The Risks of SOCIAL MEDIA

SOCIAL MEDIA *Addiction*

Bradley Steffens

ReferencePoint Press®

San Diego, CA

ReferencePoint Press®

About the Author

Bradley Steffens is a poet, a novelist, and an award-winning author of more than fifty nonfiction books for children and young adults.

Printed in the United States

For more information, contact:
ReferencePoint Press, Inc.
PO Box 27779
San Diego, CA 92198
www.ReferencePointPress.com

Picture Credits:

Cover: Shutterstock
6: FatCamera/Shutterstock
10: Maury Aaseng
12: Sam Worldey/Shutterstock
16: Depositphotos
21: SDI Productions/iStock
25: Marko Aliaksaandr/Shutterstock
27: Andrey_Popov/Shutterstock
31: Monkey Business Images/Shutterstock
34: Depositphotos
39: fizkes/Shutterstock
45: Photographee.eu/Shutterstock
48: Merla/Shutterstock
53: Ron Sachs/CNO/Newscom

LIBRARY OF CONGRESS CATALOGING-IN-PUBLICATION DATA

Names: Steffens, Bradley, 1955- author.
Title: Social media addiction / by Bradley Steffens.
Description: San Diego, CA : ReferencePoint Press, Inc., 2020. | Series: The risks of social media | Includes bibliographical references and index.
Identifiers: LCCN 2019049316 | ISBN 9781682828519 (library binding) | ISBN 9781682828526 (ebook)
Subjects: LCSH: Social media addiction.
Classification: LCC RC569.5.I54 S745 2020 | DDC 616.85/84--dc23
LC record available at https://lccn.loc.gov/2019049316

Contents

A Crisis in the Making

"I have a problem. I'm completely consumed by the urge to check all the social media platforms I occupy pretty much every minute of the day and it's destroying my entire existence," says Chrissa Hardy, a senior editor with the personal finance blog *Wise Bread*.

> "It's the same rotation every time. I hit up Instagram first, to check out my likes. Then maybe I'll scan through a celeb's feed, then 10 minutes will go by before I notice that I'm on some stranger's vacation photos from a year ago and wondering if they're still dating that other person I also don't know. My next stop is Twitter. I scroll through rage-filled political tweets to start my morning, see if any new trolls need to be blocked and then I'm on to Facebook. I share a few news stories there, some killer feminist or Game of Thrones memes and then I'm done. This is all [done] right when I wake up, BTW, and I do it at least 50 more times throughout the day without even realizing how long I spend scrolling. That's a lot of time wasted that I'll never get back. When I'm constantly scrolling, I'm not working. I should be working

during my workdays and not checking social media. On the weekends, I should be sleeping or eating or doing literally anything other than looking at my phone. And even when I can cut my time on social media down to a few minutes, it's the FOMO [fear of missing out] that keeps my mind occupied, and has me coming back again and again."[1]

Behavioral Addiction

The behavior Hardy describes is commonly referred to as social media addiction. It is a behavioral addiction that some psychologists believe is similar to gambling disorder, gaming addiction, and shopping addiction. A behavioral addiction is a mental health condition in which a person repeatedly engages in a particular behavior, even if the behavior causes him or her harm. The medical community has not officially recognized social media addiction as a psychological disorder. Many psychologists, though, have written about the problems that individuals face when overusing social media. In Hardy's case, her continual use of social media is having a negative impact on her work. It is also causing her to feel anxious.

> "I'm completely consumed by the urge to check all the social media platforms I occupy pretty much every minute of the day and it's destroying my entire existence."[1]
>
> —Chrissa Hardy, senior editor at *Wise Bread*, a personal finance blog

Mark D. Griffiths, the first psychologist to publish research recognizing the harms associated with social media addiction, defines it as occurring when the excessive use of social media damages personal, family, or professional life. Griffiths has identified six components of behavioral addiction. These include salience, when a behavior becomes a most important part of a person's life; mood modification, when a person uses a behavior to alter his or her moods or escape from problems; tolerance, when a person has to spend more time engaged in a behavior to produce the same feelings of well-being;

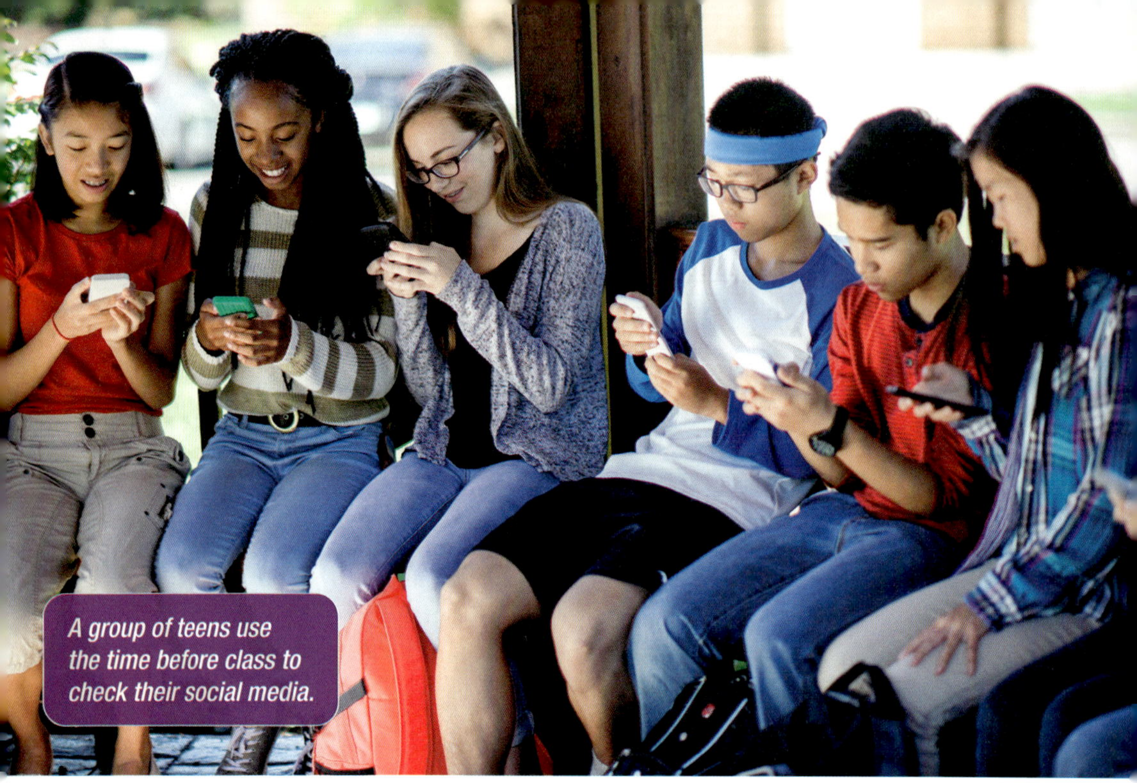

A group of teens use the time before class to check their social media.

withdrawal symptoms, when a person has unpleasant feelings or physical sensations when not able to engage in a behavior; conflict, when a behavior creates relationship problems or disrupts everyday life; and relapse, when a person tries to curb or give up a behavior but reverts to excessive use. Griffiths states that any behavior, including using social media, that fulfills these six criteria can be defined as an addiction.

The Effects of Social Media Addiction

Social media addiction has serious effects on mental health. Many heavy social media users experience severe anxiety. Hardy is one of them. "I have zero shame when talking about my anxiety," says Hardy. "I take medication for it, and I've become very familiar with my triggers in order to do my best to stay balanced. Social media makes it worse, though. It's a lot of chatter, a lot of hatred and a lot of fake BS that I don't need in my life anyway. Why am I doing this to myself?"[2]

Excessive social media use has been linked to other mental conditions as well. These include depression, loneliness, and problems with mental functioning. Researchers at Michigan State University have found that heavy users of social networking websites display signs of impaired decision-making that are similar to those of people who abuse substances such as heroin, cocaine, or methamphetamine.

Social media addiction has physical effects as well. A study by the University of Toronto found that sitting for eight to twelve hours a day, as many social media addicts do, is linked to heart disease, cancer, and early death, even if the person exercises regularly. Because users have a fear of missing out on the latest updates and trending topics, social media addiction can also affect the length and quality of their sleep. Sleep deprivation is a risk factor for several diseases, including obesity, diabetes, cardiovascular disease, and depression.

A Widespread Problem

As researchers look into the causes of anxiety and depression, they are finding more and more cases linked to social media overuse. The number of people addicted to social media worldwide is staggering, according to researchers at the University of Michigan, Flint (UMF). They found that 6 percent of the world's social media users—about 210 million people—are addicted to social networking. With more than 144 million social media users in the United States, the UMF estimate would mean that more than 8.6 million Americans are addicted to social media.

Social media addiction is a relatively new phenomenon, and its risks are only beginning to be understood. Griffiths, for example, published his initial research in 2011, but has continued to publish studies on the behavior. As its symptoms, side effects, and hazards become better known, social media addiction may be recognized by the American Psychological Association as a mental disorder, and perhaps then steps to curb its spread will be taken. Meanwhile, more and more people will occupy their days compulsively scrolling to keep up with the glut of news, pictures, memes, videos, and gossip that continually fills social media platforms.

The Scope of Social Media Addiction

According to the July 2019 report *Digital 2019: Q3 Global Digital Statshot* by internet research firms We Are Social and Hootsuite, 3.5 billion people—59 percent of the world's population over the age of thirteen—use social media. Even if a small number of these social media users are compulsive users, the population of social media addicts is enormous. If researchers at the University of Michigan are correct and an estimated 210 million people are addicted to social media worldwide, then taken together they would form the sixth-largest country in the world.

Who Is Most at Risk?

Not all countries share the same number of habitual users, though. The percentage of Americans using social media, for example, is higher than the global average. According to We Are Social and Hootsuite, 70 percent of Americans—230 million people—use social media, and most use it a lot. A July 2019 survey by Pew Research Center found that the vast majority of Americans go online several times a day, and a significant number of people—28 percent—say they are online "almost constantly." Much of this time is spent on social media sites. The rate is even higher among young adults. Roughly half of eighteen- to twenty-nine-year-olds (48 percent) say they go online almost constantly—a rate that rose 9 percentage points between 2018 and 2019. Not all heavy social media users are addicted to social media, but they might be in danger of becoming so as the years go by and the habit of constantly checking their accounts becomes ingrained in their lives.

Writer Carrie Battan admits that her interest in social media has become an addictive obsession. The amount of time she spends on social media has been a source of friction between her and her partner. As a result, she sometimes hides her activity from him. "I am . . . constantly searching for down moments with my partner during which to check my phone," she says.

> **"Sometimes I will catch myself lingering in the bathroom for an extra 20 minutes . . . idly scrolling through my social media feeds like a sugar addict digging through a pile of empty candy wrappers hoping to find scraps."[3]**
>
> — Carrie Battan, writer and social media addict

> Sometimes I will catch myself lingering in the bathroom for an extra 20 minutes after I've brushed my teeth, idly scrolling through my social media feeds like a sugar addict digging through a pile of empty candy wrappers hoping to find scraps. "What were you doing?" my partner will ask when I've emerged, accusatorially. I can't even tell him, because I don't know.[3]

Teens are at a higher risk of social media addiction than are adults like Battan. A June 2018 survey by Pew Research found that social media use is nearly ubiquitous among today's teens. Fully 97 percent of 13- to 17-year-olds use at least one of seven major online platforms. An astounding 45 percent of teens say they are online almost constantly. This is a major concern to psychologists, because the adolescent prefrontal cortex—the part of the brain that is responsible for functions such as judgment, decision-making, problem solving, and impulse control—does not

Nearly Half of Young Adults Are Online Almost Constantly

Nearly half of US adults age eighteen to twenty-nine say they are online "almost constantly," according to a 2019 Pew Research Center poll. A significant number of slightly older adults (between thirty and forty-nine years old) also spend a lot of time online. Experts say that much of this time is spent on social media sites. Although this does not automatically translate to addiction, it may indicate a developing dependence or addiction.

Roughly three in ten Americans—and 48 percent of those ages 18–29—go online "almost constantly"

Percent of US adults in each group who say they go online "almost constantly"

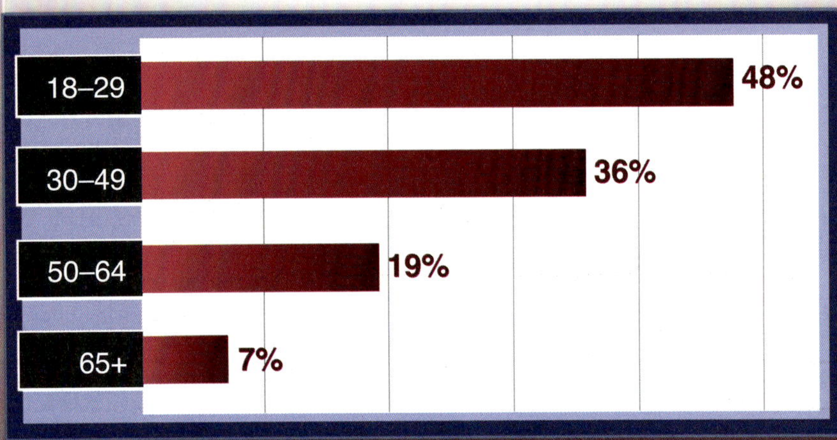

Source: Andrew Perrin and Madhu Kumar, "About Three-in-Ten U.S. Adults Say They Are 'Almost Constantly' Online," Pew Research Center, July 25, 2019. www.pewresearch.org.

fully mature until a person reaches his or her twenties. Without a fully developed ability to control their actions, teens are more prone to succumb to their urges to check their social media accounts. "I think they're addicted to the peer connection and affirmation they're able to get via social media," says clinical child psychologist Marion Underwood. "To know what each other are doing, where they stand, to know how many people like what they posted, to know how many people followed them today and unfollowed them . . . that I think is highly addictive."[4]

A 2016 study by researchers at the University of Bergen in Norway found that young people were more susceptible to the affirmation and interaction offered on social media than older people. This finding was not surprising, write the researchers, because the younger generation "often uses such technologies in order to acquire, develop and maintain relationships, and may seek feedback on their behaviors and online persona as a way of forming and/or enhancing their social identity."[5] While using technology to form relationships is not necessarily a problem, it can be when the urge for seeking feedback becomes an obsession. "The most times I check it (my phone) in a day? I lose track. It's just a need," one teen told CNN. "Even though I was at school, I would still check my phone because I mean, people post things at school and stuff, so you still always worry."[6] An Italian student who took part in a global challenge to give up all internet activity for just one day found that she was extremely anxious without social media and other online contact. "I am not receiving messages, photos, emails, likes, comments, etc.," she says. "It feels as if no one is willing to interact with me, thinking about me! I am alone!!"[7]

> **"I think [teens are] addicted to the peer connection and affirmation they're able to get via social media."[4]**
>
> — Marion Underwood, clinical child psychologist

Teen girls are at greater risk of social media addiction than teen boys are. The Pew Research Center reports that girls are more likely than boys to say that they spend too much time on social media—47 percent to 35 percent. "Social media is girl town," says Rachel Simmons, author of *Odd Girl Out: The Hidden Culture of Aggression in Girls*. "They are all over it in ways that boys are not." Not only are girls more exposed to social media, but Simmons and others believe girls also are more concerned with what their peers think of them. Social media plays on these insecurities, according to Simmons. "It used to be that you didn't know how many friends someone had, or what they were doing after school," Simmons says. "Social media assigns numbers to those things. For the most vulnerable girls, that can be very destabilizing."[8]

Teens in general feel anxious about the images of themselves that they present through social media. "I definitely feel pressure to look perfect on Instagram," another female teen told CNN. "What goes through my mind as I'm posting a picture about myself is—I'm thinking, 'What will people think of this? Are they going to approve? Are they going to think I'm ugly, are they going to think I'm pretty?' I'm thinking all these things and I'm comparing myself to others."[9] If social media users do not get the expected or desired response, they can feel additional anxiety. "I'm nervous about what people think and are going to say," says a teen named Athena. "It sometimes bugs me when I don't get a certain amount of likes on a picture."[10]

People with low self-esteem are also at greater risk of developing a social media addiction, according to the University of Bergen study. In fact, low self-esteem is the greatest of all risk factors found in the study. "After controlling for all other variables in the equation, low self-esteem had the strongest effect on addictive social media use, followed by being a woman,"[11] write the researchers. Cecilie Schou Andreassen, a professor of psychology at the University of Bergen, describes the connection between low self-esteem and social media addiction: "Cognitions [thoughts] activate behavior,

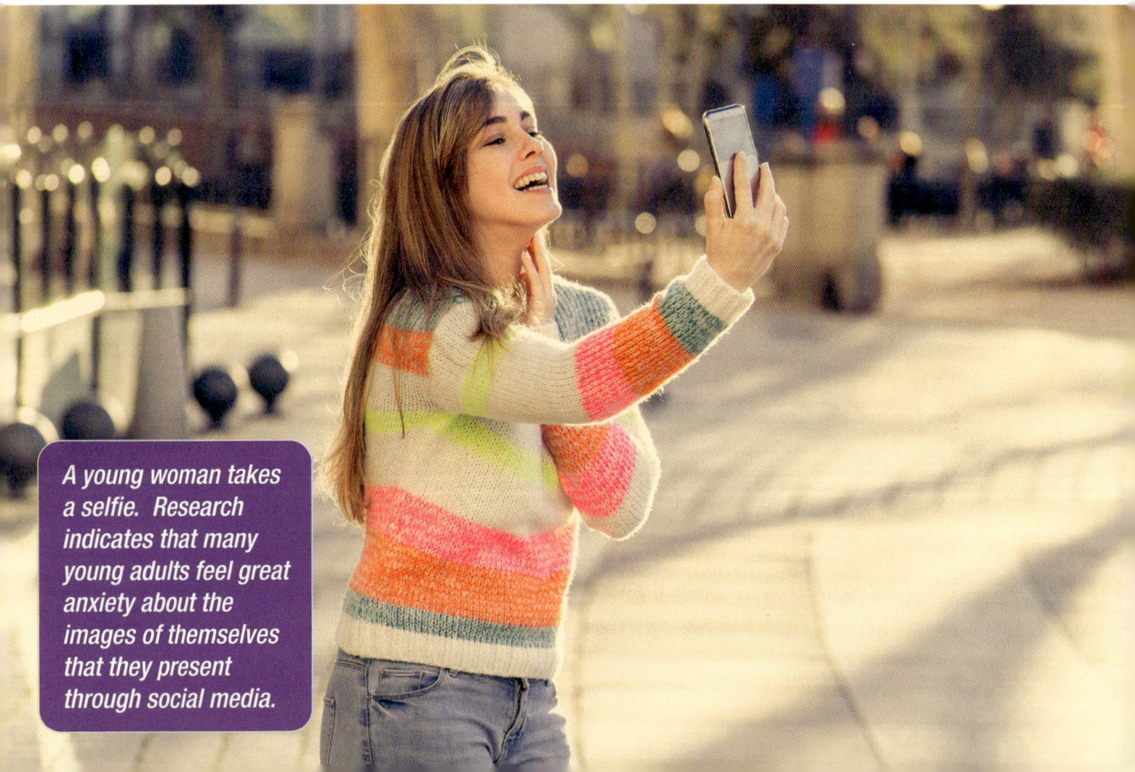

A young woman takes a selfie. Research indicates that many young adults feel great anxiety about the images of themselves that they present through social media.

and may therefore activate social networking behavior. A negative self-concept ('I'm not good enough' or 'I lack social skills') may trigger social networking behavior in cases where the person believes number of 'likes' and 'followers' on a [social networking site] equals success, and leads to compulsive social networking."[12]

The Lure of Social Media

One of the reasons why social media is so popular is that it offers many different activities that appeal to different interests. People who want to keep up with what their friends are doing can view their activities on Facebook. Those who want to read what people they respect and admire are saying can do so on Twitter. Others who like to look at pictures of friends, celebrities, and other interesting people can do so on Instagram or Snapchat. Users who enjoy videos can watch them on YouTube. And these are just the most popular social media sites: there are many more, including interactive blogs, message boards, and forums. Even online gaming is considered a form of social media when gamers play mainly to speak or chat with other players. Social media includes something for almost everyone.

The variety of things to do on social media sites contributes to addiction, according to researchers at the University of Lancaster in England and the University of Bamberg in Germany. These experts found that when social media users experience stress on a social media site, they cope with the stress by moving from one activity to another, rather than by leaving the site or logging off the internet. "Because social network sites offer such a wide range of features, users can find they act both as stressors and as a distraction from that stress,"[13] observes Christian Maier, assistant professor of information systems at the University of Bamberg and a coauthor of the study. For example, Facebook users might switch from scanning their news feed to chatting with friends, or from chatting with friends to posting an update, when each activity begins to cause stress. The researchers found that the more that individuals use social media, the more likely it is that they will stay within the social networking site rather than leaving it when they need to divert themselves. The

Warning Signs of Social Media Addiction

Sarah Fader, the chief executive officer (CEO) and founder of Stigma Fighters, a nonprofit organization that encourages individuals with mental illness to share their personal stories, provides a list of the most common symptoms of social media addiction:

- Interrupting conversations to check your social media accounts
- Lying to others about how much time you spend on social media
- Withdrawal from friends and family
- Trying to stop or reduce your use of social media more than once before without being successful
- Loss of interest in other activities
- Neglecting work or school to comment on Facebook or Twitter account
- Experiencing withdrawal symptoms when you are not able to access social media
- Spending over six hours per day on social networking sites like Facebook, Twitter, or Instagram
- Overwhelming need to share things with others on social media sites
- Having your phone with you 24 hours a day to check your social media sites
- Using social media more often than you planned
- Severe nervousness or anxiety when you are not able to check your notifications
- Negative impacts in your personal or professional life due to social media usage

Sarah Fader, "Social Media Obsession and Anxiety," Anxiety and Depression Association of America, November 2019. https://adaa.org.

users who spend the greatest amount of time on social media are the most likely to keep using it to cope with the stress it creates. The researchers believe this cycle of behavior is one of the factors that leads to social media addiction.

Using social media to relieve the stress caused by social media rarely works. Since the users do not leave the social networking site, they continue to feel anxiety. The longer they are on the social networking site, the more anxiety they feel. They can get locked into a downward spiral of anxiety, compulsion, and finally addiction. Says Maier:

> Even when users are stressed from [social networking site] use, they are using the same platforms to cope with that stress, diverting themselves through other activities on the [social networking site], and ultimately building compulsive and excessive behaviour. As a result, they embed themselves in the social network environment rather than getting away from it, and an addiction is formed.[14]

Underlying Mental Disorders

People with mental disorders are also at high risk of becoming addicted to social media. Social media addiction is mainly a matter of impulse control, and impaired impulse control is a symptom of various mental disorders that may exist before a person goes online or becomes interested in social media. For example, attention-deficit/hyperactivity disorder (ADHD) is characterized by a lack of impulse control. When a person with ADHD goes online, his or her impaired impulse control can contribute not only to social media addiction, but also to gaming addiction, shopping addiction, or online gambling addiction. Other disorders can also contribute to social media addiction. These include anxiety disorders, mood disorders, behavioral disorders, and autism spectrum disorder (ASD).

> "Even when users are stressed from [social media] use, they are using the same platforms to cope with that stress, diverting themselves through other activities on [these sites], and ultimately building compulsive and excessive behaviour."[14]
>
> — Christian Maier, assistant professor of information systems at the University of Bamberg

Scientists at DePaul University's College of Computing and Digital Media have found that some heavy users of social media have a deficiency in the part of the brain that governs impulse control. Human beings have two different mechanisms in their brain that influence their decision-making. One system, known as the cognitive-emotional preoccupation system, is automatic and reactive. It reacts quickly to outside stimulation, such as a sight of food, facial expressions, or even notifications from social media. The second system, known as the cognitive-behavioral control system, is reflective and guided by reason. It responds more slowly to stimulation, which includes thoughts generated by the first system. This system helps individuals control impulses and behaviors that are not in their best interest. Both systems are essential to survival, one to make quick decisions and the other to make more thoughtful ones.

The DePaul University researchers found that individuals who use Facebook excessively have a strong cognitive-emotional preoccupation system and a weak cognitive-behavioral control system. The greater the imbalance between the two systems, the more likely individuals were to engage in excessive social media use, and the greater the risk that they would become addicted to social media.

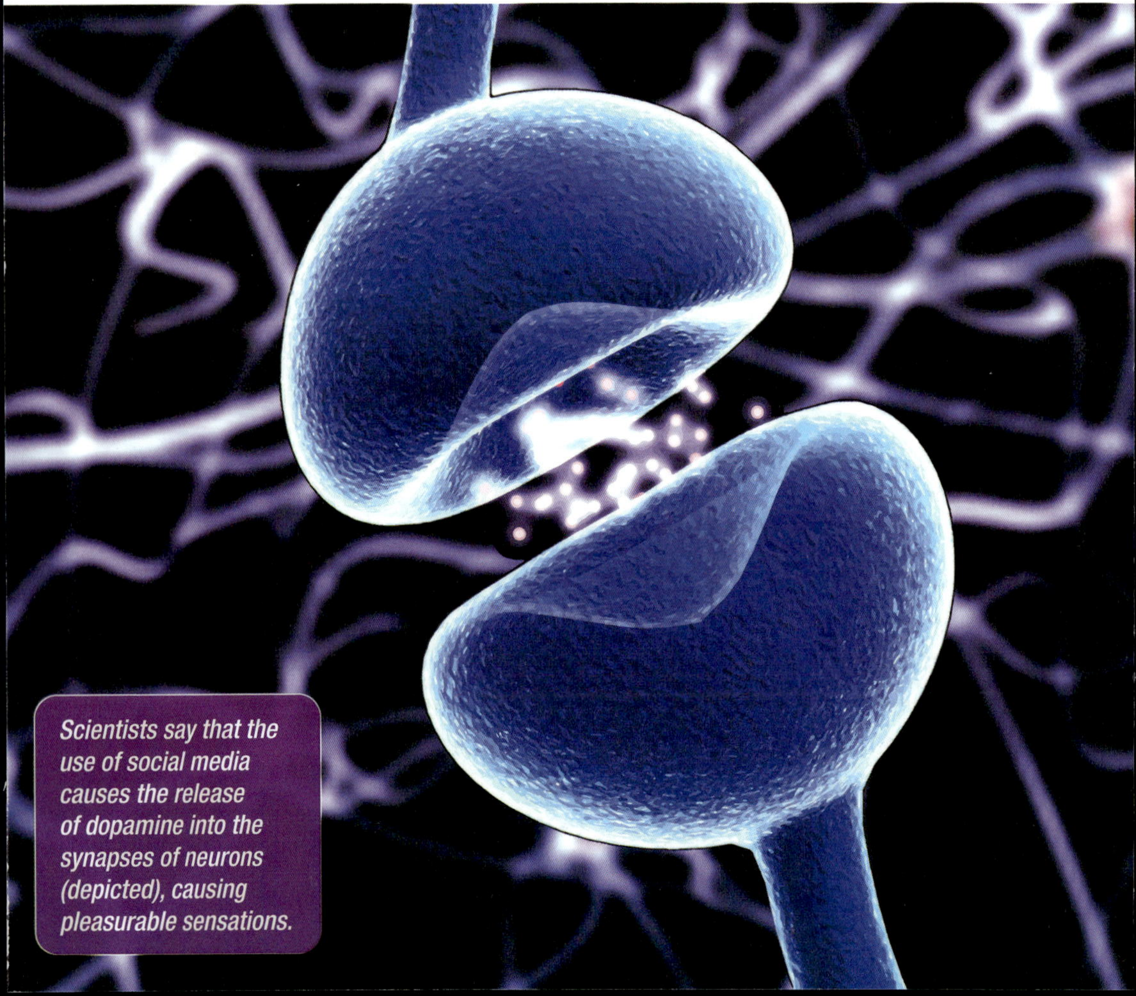

Scientists say that the use of social media causes the release of dopamine into the synapses of neurons (depicted), causing pleasurable sensations.

A Journalist Recognizes Her Social Media Addiction

Hayley Sewell, a reporter for BusinessCloud, a technology news website, describes her social media addiction:

> How many times do you look at your mobile phone a day? I checked my usage levels recently and apparently I look at mine nearly 100 times every day. . . .
>
> I should have realised the overpowering nature of my addiction when I checked my Facebook while watching a film at the cinema. It wasn't a very good film but that's no excuse. . . .
>
> I find myself in a social media hole at times—opening each one in rotation, looking for new content and moving on to the next. By the time I'm back around to the beginning, enough time has passed for new content, and so it continues. It's a dangerous cycle, especially before bed. . . .
>
> [Social media] makes us feel connected and almost special, which millennials have been branded as our problem—we want to feel noticed in this big world. . . .
>
> I've never smoked but I imagine I'm addicted to social media like smokers crave nicotine. I've resolved to cut back but I'm honest enough to know that I couldn't stop completely.

Hayley Sewell, "My Social Media Addiction Took Over My Life," *BusinessCloud*, February 4, 2019. www.businesscloud.co.uk.

A Need to Share

Beyond stimulating cognitive control systems, social media connects to a deep human need that most people are not even aware of: a need to share information about oneself. Researchers Diana I. Tamir and Jason P. Mitchell used magnetic resonance imaging to explore brain activity when people talk about themselves. They found that when people discuss themselves, they experience a pleasant feeling, similar to the natural rewards that accompany eating. This is because self-disclosure activates the brain regions that release dopamine, the body's natural, pleasure-giving reward substance. The reaction was so strong that the research subjects were willing to pass up money in order to disclose information about themselves. The researchers found that this desire for self-exposure begins very early in a person's life.

Based on their tests, Tamir and Mitchell concluded that human beings have an intrinsic, or in-born, drive for self-exposure. Social networking sites give an outlet to this deep human drive, and a user's brain is rewarded with dopamine for sharing personal information; and when that information is "liked" or commented upon, the pleasure is compounded. "People dedicate close to 40% of their time talking about themselves," write the researchers. "This number reaches 80% in social networks with the possibility of feedback and immediate rewards."[15]

The existence of a deep-seated need to share information is one reason why social media is popular around the world, regardless of country, language, or culture. The rewards the brain gives social media users for sharing information about themselves makes involvement with social media a pleasurable experience. For many people, the allure of social media is difficult to resist and can grow into an obsession. "Technological addiction can happen to anyone,"[16] says digital addiction expert Holland Haiis.

Chapter Two

Why People Become Addicted to Social Media

The fact that some people become addicted to social media is no accident. It is by design. Social media sites are big business. The companies that operate them earn money from advertisers based on how many people view advertisements in the social media stream. Keeping users engaged with the social media site increases the number of ads that are seen and the amount of money the social media site earns. As a result, social media companies do everything they can to keep their users engaged with their sites. This includes an array of techniques developed by the gambling industry, the advertising industry, and their own research. These techniques trigger reactions in the brain that can be addictive. "You have a business model designed to engage you and get you to basically suck as much time out of your life as possible and then selling that attention to advertisers," says former Facebook engineer Sandy Parakilas. "There was definitely an awareness of the fact that the product was habit-forming and addictive."[17]

Activating a Natural Reward System

Researchers and executives who work in industries that prosper from certain behaviors, including the advertising, gambling, and social media industries, have a deep knowledge of how the human brain works. They use this knowledge to shape behavior, manipulating people without their ever knowing it. For example, social media executives know that dopamine creates a pleasant sensation and feeling of well-being. All mammals, including humans, produce dopamine. In a natural state, dopamine promotes survival by rewarding the animal or person with a pleasant sensation when the living thing does something that helps ensure survival, such as eating, drinking, or procreating. In the modern world, people can release dopamine by succeeding at challenges, such as winning a tennis match or solving a puzzle. Creating a popular post on a social media website can also release dopamine. The effect is literally intoxicating. "In terms of drugs, we know that the faster something reaches your brain, the more addicting it is, since it lights up your brain's reward system so quickly," says Erin Vogel, a postdoctoral psychiatry fellow at the University of California, San Francisco. "Social media engagement is instantaneous; you upload a photo, you get validation, you want more."[18]

The release of dopamine is more complicated than it might seem, however. For one thing, the brain has to know that the person has done something well. If a person posts a picture on Facebook that many people enjoy, that alone will not release dopamine. The person who posted the picture needs to know that other people enjoyed it. This is why social media designers created rewards systems for users. Justin Rosenstein, a former Facebook engineer, created the "like" button so users could show their appreciation for posts, and so the person who created the post could be rewarded. Rosenstein calls these rewards "bright dings of pseudo-pleasure,"[19] because they cause the brain to release dopamine, creating a brief feeling of well-being.

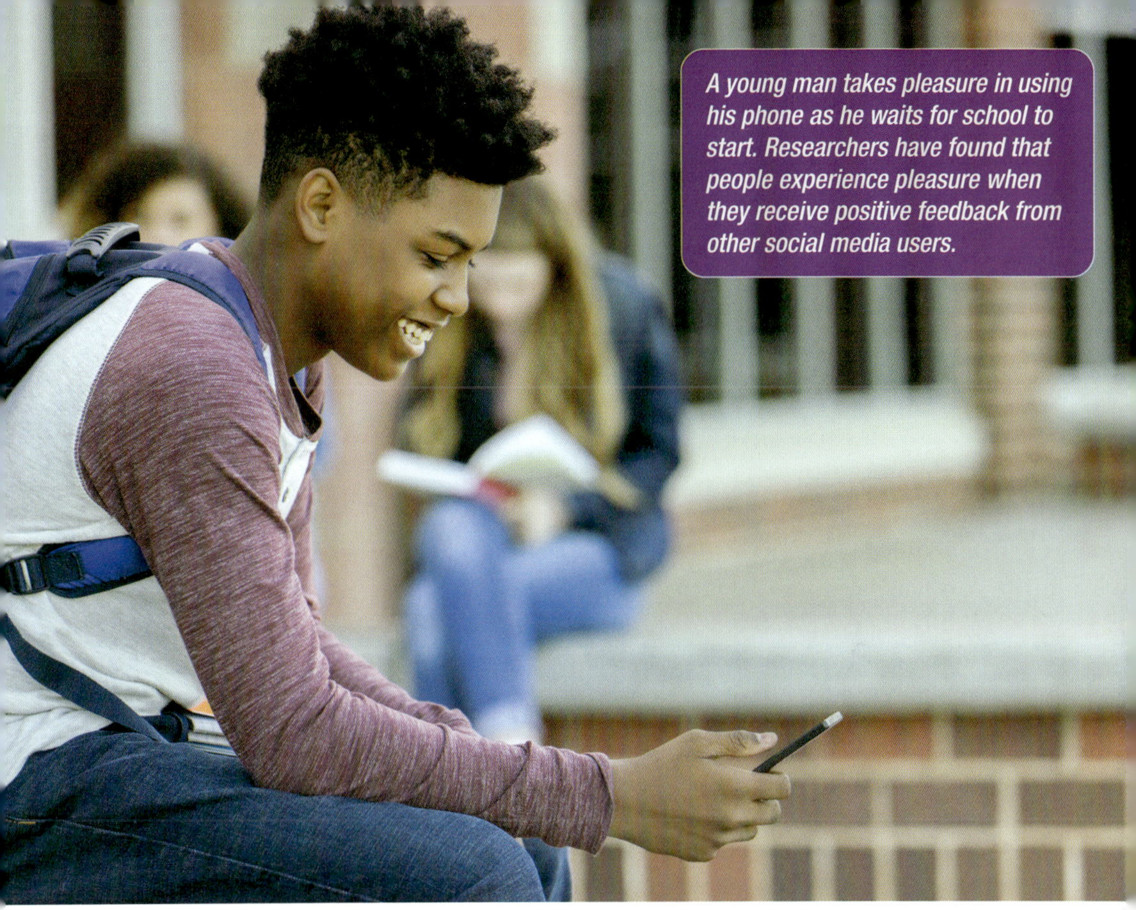

A young man takes pleasure in using his phone as he waits for school to start. Researchers have found that people experience pleasure when they receive positive feedback from other social media users.

The brain does not release dopamine for every feat, however. If it did, people would be in a constant state of bliss, and that would not help ensure survival. Feeling contented, they would stop seeking the next meal, the next drink of water, or the solution to the next problem. The brain only releases dopamine when a successful outcome follows a period of uncertainty, as when an animal succeeds in a hunt after following a scent.

Creating Uncertainty

The feedback mechanisms in social media mimic the periods of uncertainty that occur naturally. The person who posts a picture or a statement in Facebook, Twitter, or Instagram does not know how many "likes," "loves," "shares," "retweets," or comments the item will receive, and whether the feedback will be positive or negative. This uncertainty fuels the dopamine release when positive feedback is received.

This system behind this uncertainty is known as "intermittent variable rewards." It is the same technique used to keep gamblers playing slot machines, when the pull of a lever may result in one of a range of prizes or nothing at all. Curiosity about the reaction of others and the anticipation of a reward keep people hooked on social media, the way gamblers get hooked on playing slot machines. "The rewards are what psychologists refer to as variable reinforcement schedules and is the key to social media users repeatedly checking their screens,"[20] says Mark Griffiths, a professor of behavioral addiction and director of Nottingham Trent University's International Gaming Research Unit. Users anticipate positive reactions—reinforcement—to their posts, so they keep posting and checking their posts. The schedule of that reinforcement is variable because users never know when the reactions might come. "Social media sites are chock-a-block with unpredictable rewards," says Griffiths. "They are trying to grab users' attentions . . . to make social media users create a routine and habitually check their screens."[21] For some social media users, intermittent variable rewards stimulate their interest to the point of addictiveness.

"Social media sites are chock-a-block with unpredictable rewards. They are trying to grab users' attentions . . . to make social media users create a routine and habitually check their screens."[21]

—Mark Griffiths, professor of behavioral addiction at Nottingham Trent University

Hooked on Rewards

The variable rewards that writer Shaun Smith received for his posts on Twitter turned him into a social media addict. "I started my journey on social media in the spring of 2018 on Twitter," says Smith. "As soon as one of my early tweets received a few likes and interactions I was hooked and hopelessly lost down the rabbit hole of social media addiction." He tweeted about parenting using hashtags like #dadlife, #momsquad, and #parenting, which brought him to the attention of like-minded Twitter users. "As it

Social Media Disorder Scale Survey

The Social Media Disorder Scale is a nine-question survey developed in 2016 by Regina J. J. M. van der Eijnden, a researcher at Utrecht University in the Netherlands, to distinguish between healthy and unhealthy social media use. A person taking the survey simply gives a *yes* or *no* answer to each of the questions. Five or more *yes* answers meet the criteria for a formal diagnosis of a disordered social media user.

During the past year, have you . . .

. . . regularly found that you can't think of anything else but the moment that you will be able to use social media again?

. . . regularly felt dissatisfied because you wanted to spend more time on social media?

. . . often felt bad when you could not use social media?

. . . tried to spend less time on social media, but failed?

. . . regularly neglected other activities (e.g. hobbies, sport) because you wanted to use social media?

. . . regularly had arguments with others because of your social media use?

. . . regularly lied to your parents or friends about the amount of time you spend on social media?

. . . often used social media to escape from negative feelings?

. . . had serious conflict with your parents, brother(s) or sister(s) because of your social media use?

Center for Research on Children, Adolescents, and the Media, "Social Media Disorder Scale (SMD Scale)," 2019. www.ccam-ascor.nl.

turned out I was fairly good at writing and sharing my parenting humor and I quickly became twitter 'famous' sort of speaking," Smith recalls. Soon his tweets were being featured in various parenting blogs and even popular websites like BuzzFeed and Babble. "I even went 'viral' multiple times over," he says. "I was enjoying the ride and the rush I'd get from all the attention."[22]

Smith became obsessed with repeating his successes.

> I'd find myself checking notifications, always forming my next joke in my head and rushing to get it written down before I forgot it. My addiction got so bad that even my oldest daughter started calling me "Mr. Twitter" and "Twitter man." That should have been eye opening enough to make me scale back my social media usage, but it wasn't. I tried to put the phone down, but I was pulled to the instant ability to chat and interact with hundreds of other parents. The ability to share my stories, jokes, failures and wins as a father was too much for me to resist.[23]

Smith realized that he was in the grips of an addiction.

> When people "like" or "share" or "comment" on what you've posted you feel happy as if they agree with you. When this happens your brain cells stimulate dopamine and this makes you feel good and happy. This is one of the main reasons causing the addiction. The "notifications" going off on my phone were my drug and I craved them day and night.[24]

After ten months of building up his Twitter following, Smith's wife confronted him about his preoccupation with social media. She said that she felt like a bystander in their relationship. "It's as though you don't exist anymore and none of us matter to you," she told him. Her words got through to him. "On that day I finally saw and realized all the damage I had done to her and to us," says Smith. He deactivated his Twitter account that day and did not go back. "I'm still rebuilding our relationship back to where it was pre-addiction," he says. "Social media addiction is new, it's real, it ruins relationships and I'm a recovering addict."[25]

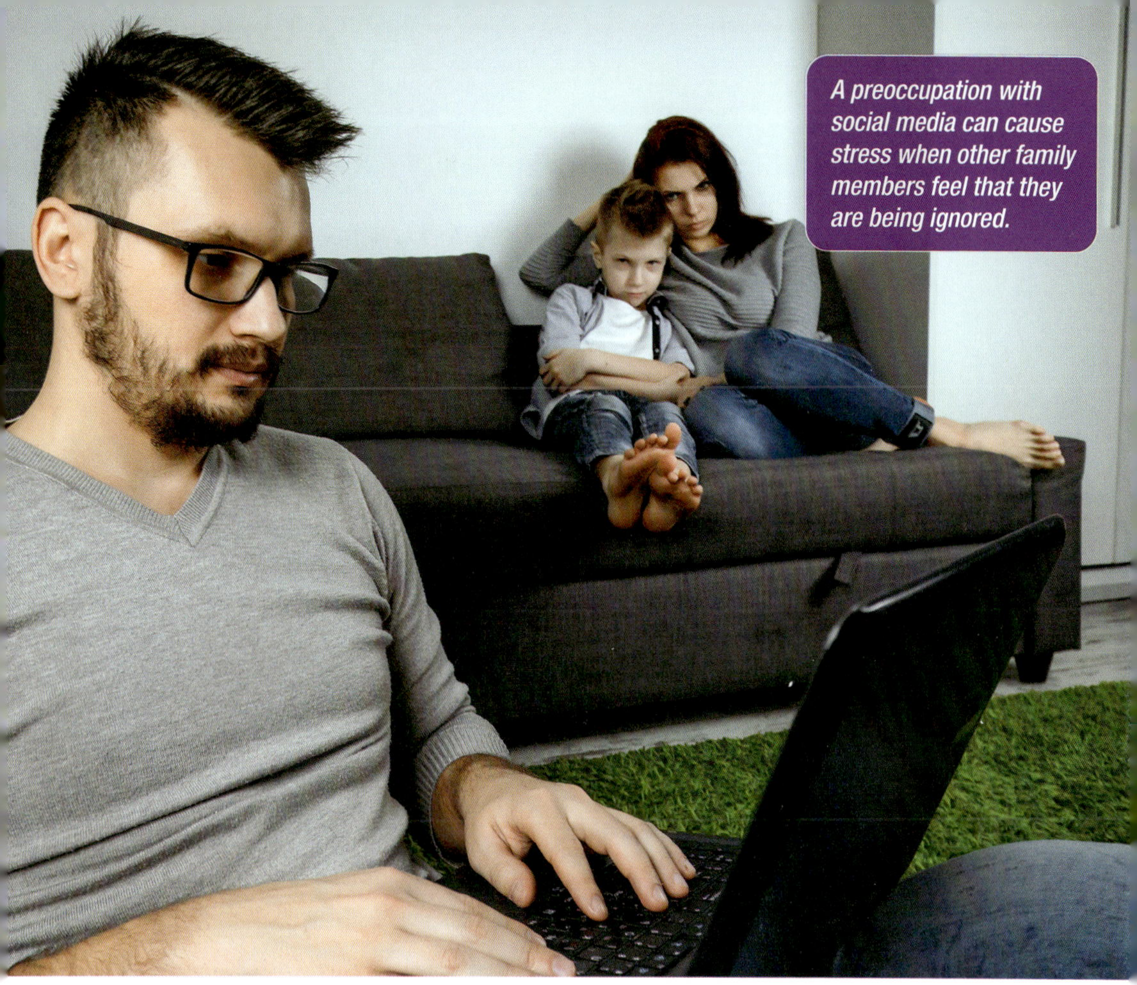

A preoccupation with social media can cause stress when other family members feel that they are being ignored.

An Endless Loop

Social media rewards do not necessarily end when the user sees the likes and comments on their posts. Many people feel obligated to respond to the comments they receive by making comments of their own. Responding to feedback keeps users on the sites even longer, exactly as designed. "All of us are jacked into this system," says Tristan Harris, a former Google employee. "All of our minds can be hijacked. Our choices are not as free as we think they are."[26]

To make sure people are aware of the feedback they are receiving, social media sites send out messages or notifications every time a post or comment has been liked or commented on. Curious about the notifications, many users check them immediately to see what was liked or said. These notifications draw the user back to the social media site. "It's as if they're taking behavioral cocaine and just sprinkling it all over your interface," says Aza Raskin, a software engineer who invented the feature that allows users to scroll indefinitely on any social media site. "And that's the thing that keeps you like coming back and back and back." Raskin says that social media companies are constantly testing new features to make them ever more alluring. "Behind every screen on your phone, there are generally like literally a thousand (user experience) engineers that have worked on this thing to try to make it maximally addicting,"[27] he says.

Dana Chisnell, codirector of the Center for Civic Design, a nonprofit organization devoted to improve the voting experience, feels manipulated by the strategies employed by social media sites. "Being online all the time is stressful and distracting," she says. "It has come to feel like I'm performing for the makers of the platform rather than having real conversations. There are too many channels running concurrently, and it's too hard to keep up. I feel unfocused all the time."[28]

> **"Being online all the time is stressful and distracting. It has come to feel like I'm performing for the makers of the platform rather than having real conversations."[28]**
>
> — Dana Chisnell, codirector of the Center for Civic Design

Social media sites also send out a notification every time a person receives a message, causing the user's device to light up with a notification and to make a noise, such as a chime (unless this feature is turned off). Many users feel an urgency to respond to messages and notifications. A survey by Common Sense Media finds that 48 percent of adults and 72 percent of teens feel obligated to respond immediately to texts, social networking messages, and notifications. The habit of immediately responding to social media alerts further increases the amount of time spent in the sites and causes disruption in the user's life. "Too many of us have become slaves to the devices that were supposed to free us," says Jane E. Brody, a columnist for the *New York Times*. "Instead, we're constantly bombarded by bells,

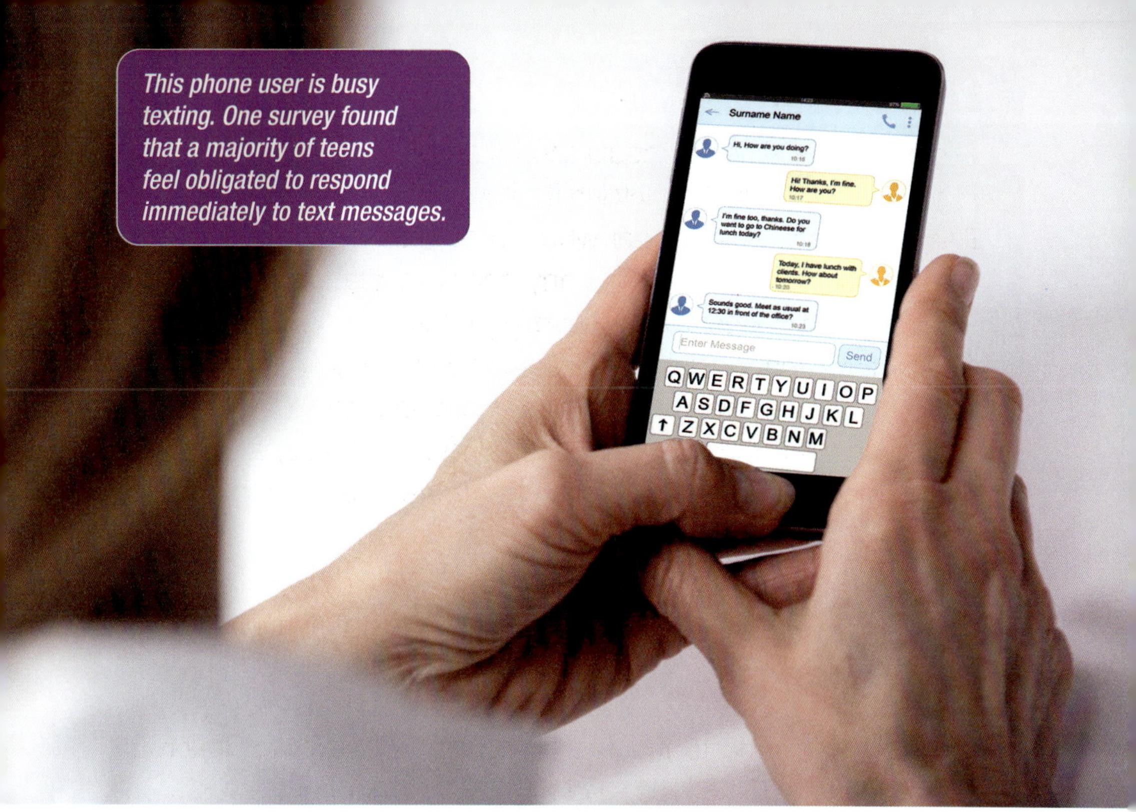

This phone user is busy texting. One survey found that a majority of teens feel obligated to respond immediately to text messages.

buzzers and chimes that alert us to messages we feel compelled to view and respond to immediately."[29]

If a person uses several social media sites, the number of notifications is multiplied. This is the case for many Americans. While the majority of older Americans use only one or two social media websites—mainly Facebook and YouTube—the majority of young adults and teens use multiple social media sites. According to the Pew Research Center, 94 percent of eighteen- to twenty-four-year-olds use YouTube, 78 percent use Snapchat, 71 percent use Instagram, 68 percent use Facebook, and 45 percent use Twitter. With that many social media accounts, the bombardment of notifications can be endless.

The constant barrage of alerts and notifications can affect the brain on a deep level. For example, heavy users of social media sometimes think their phone is vibrating, or that they have received a message, even when they have not. "Phantom calls and notifications are linked to our psychological craving for such signals," says Daniel Kruger, a research associate professor of

A TV Personality Faces Her Social Media Addiction

Lisa Canning is an interior designer from HGTV's "Buying and Selling with the Property Brothers." In 2019, she took a thirty-day break from social media, only to find she was addicted. She writes:

> When my husband challenged me to the concept of a work and social media sabbatical for 30 days, I knew it was going to be hard. But I had no idea how hard. For the first 2 days I had literal shakes. I had removed my email, and all social media apps from my phone, but the habit of checking my social media app at any available moment had become so habitual, that I would tap the blank screen where they once were. When I would open my phone and realize there was nothing on it to do on my phone, I would sit there restless and unsettled. I had no idea how much I had relied on my social media apps to provide me affirmation, entertainment and a means of escape. Kicking the habit of constantly engaging my mind and my thumbs was a really hard shift.

Lisa Canning, "Here's What Happened When I Recognized My Social Media Addiction," *Red Tricycle*, April 17, 2019. https://redtri.com.

health behavior and health education at the University of Michigan. "These social media messages can activate the same brain mechanisms as cocaine [does]." The manipulation of the brain is not accidental, says Kruger. "There are whole departments trying to design their systems to be as addictive as possible. They want you to be permanently online and by bombarding you with messages and stimuli try to redirect your attention back to their app or webpage."[30]

Fear of Missing Out

For many social media users, ignoring notifications is not feasible. Users grow increasingly anxious when they do not check their social media accounts. Researchers call this anxiety the "fear of missing out," or "FOMO." "The FOMO experience specifically is this feeling that I personally could have been there and I wasn't," explains Amy Summerville, a professor of psychology at Miami University in Ohio. "I do think that part of the reason that's really powerful is this cue that maybe we're not being included by people we have important social relationships with."[31] People in the throes of FOMO check their social media not simply to satisfy their curiosity but to alleviate their anxiety. Engaging in a behavior to modify a person's moods, especially to relieve anxiety or other negative feelings, is the hallmark of behavioral addiction.

> **"These social media messages can activate the same brain mechanisms as cocaine [does]."[30]**
>
> — Daniel Kruger, research associate professor at the University of Michigan

When a person needs to engage in a behavior to modify his or her moods or satisfy a craving, that behavior is no longer a choice: it is a compulsion. "You let it go from being something you enjoy to something that's controlling you,"[32] says Douglas Gentile, a professor of psychology at Iowa State University. The need to engage in the behavior is so strong that it becomes more important than other life interests and daily activities. As a result, a person's relationships, education, and work suffer. This is the very definition of social media addiction.

The Effects of Social Media Addiction

According to some psychologists, social media addiction impairs personal, family, social, educational, occupational, and other important areas of functioning. The effects of social media addiction on these areas are reason enough for an individual to seek treatment for the addiction. But most experts acknowledge that the damage does not end there. Research shows that social media addiction can also affect a person's mental and physical health.

Effects on Work and Academic Performance

An obvious sign that individuals are addicted to social media is that their performance at work or in school suffers. The consequences of poor performance—bad grades, poor reviews, and even termination from a job—are often a wake-up call that forces these users to recognize they have a problem. While many individuals report that social media has harmed their effectiveness at work or school, such stories are not considered scientific proof that social media addiction impairs performance. That is because such stories, known also as anecdotes, are not part of a controlled study. A controlled study compares large numbers of people who are of similar age and background. This is done to eliminate the possibility that differences in age and background are the reason for the outcomes observed. A controlled study then compares people engaged in a certain behavior to those who are not engaged in it. This is done to ensure it is the behavior, not something else, that is producing the outcome.

In 2017, researchers at DePaul University and California State University, Fullerton, conducted a controlled study of 341 Facebook users at a major North American university to measure the effect of social media on academic performance. The students were of a similar age and background. Fifty-two percent of the subjects were women, and 48 percent were men. The researchers studied this group because university students are more prone than others to develop problematic use of social networking sites due to their flexible schedules, free time, high level of social media use, and little external control over their internet

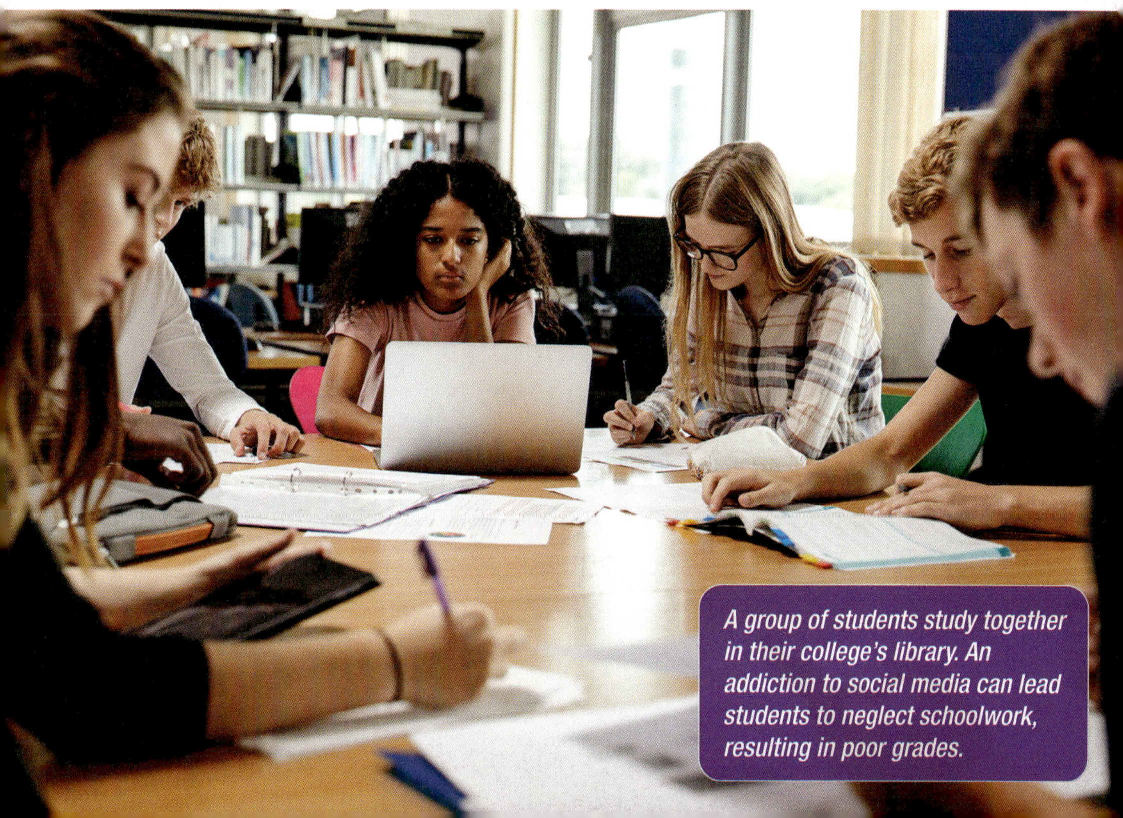

A group of students study together in their college's library. An addiction to social media can lead students to neglect schoolwork, resulting in poor grades.

habits. The researchers had the students complete two surveys at different times during the semester about their Facebook use. They found that 76 percent of respondents reported using Facebook during class, 65 percent reported using Facebook at work instead of working, 63 percent reported using Facebook while talking face-to-face with others, and 40 percent reported using Facebook while driving. Those who used Facebook in the most inappropriate and risky situations were deemed to be problematic Facebook users.

The researchers then looked at the students' grades at the end of the semester and again one year later. They found that problematic Facebook use negatively affected the students' academic performance. The greater the problematic use, the lower the students' grade point average (GPA). "The clear and strong effect of problematic social media use on an academic performance was astounding," says Ofir Turel, a professor of information systems and decision sciences at California State University, Fullerton, and a coauthor of the study. "A slight increase in problematic social media use translates into significant grade loss, and this declined performance is persistent—it remained one year after our initial study."[33]

Sleep Disruption

Problematic social media users experience a decline in GPA in part because they are distracted by social media in class, when reading and studying, and when writing research papers or completing other assignments. A contributing factor to their poor performance could also be sleep deprivation. A lack of restful sleep contributes to a lack of focus in work and study, and research shows that heavy social media use has a negative impact on sleep. In a 2018 study, researchers at the University of Glasgow in Scotland asked 101 adolescents aged twelve to eighteen years about their social media habits and sleep times. The researchers found that nighttime social media use was associated with later bedtimes, longer times to fall asleep, and shorter sleep duration.

Tolerance

Social media addicts crave the pleasant sensations provided by the release of dopamine, but these feelings can become harder and harder to achieve. Over time, the user's brain becomes so accustomed to the rewards of social media that it requires increasing amounts of them to release dopamine. This phenomenon is known as tolerance. It is one of the six criteria that Griffiths says are required for social media addiction.

Tolerance increases the user's anxiety, because it takes the user longer to achieve the mood change he or she wants and needs. As the anxiety increases, even more dopamine is required to counteract the rising tension. The release of additional dopamine takes even more time, which, in turn, causes more anxiety. For some users, tolerance is so great that their addictive behavior no longer satisfies their cravings. As a result, the social media addict can experience depression along with anxiety.

Further analysis showed that the fear of missing out predicted shorter sleep duration. There were two reasons for this relationship. The fear of missing out drives late-night social media use, which delays bedtimes. Fear of missing out also affects the person's thoughts before going to sleep, further delaying the onset of sleep. "Efforts to develop and evaluate intervention strategies should therefore consider not only social media behaviours but also underlying cognitive factors, such as fear of missing out,"[34] write the researchers.

The 2018 study confirmed the findings of a 2016 study conducted by the same researchers. The 2016 study examined how social media use related to sleep quality, self-esteem, anxiety, and depression in 467 Scottish adolescents. The researchers measured overall social media use, nighttime social media use, emotional investment in social media, sleep quality, self-esteem, and levels of anxiety and depression. They found that adolescents who used social media more—both overall and at night—and those who were more emotionally invested in social media experienced poorer sleep quality, lower self-esteem, and higher

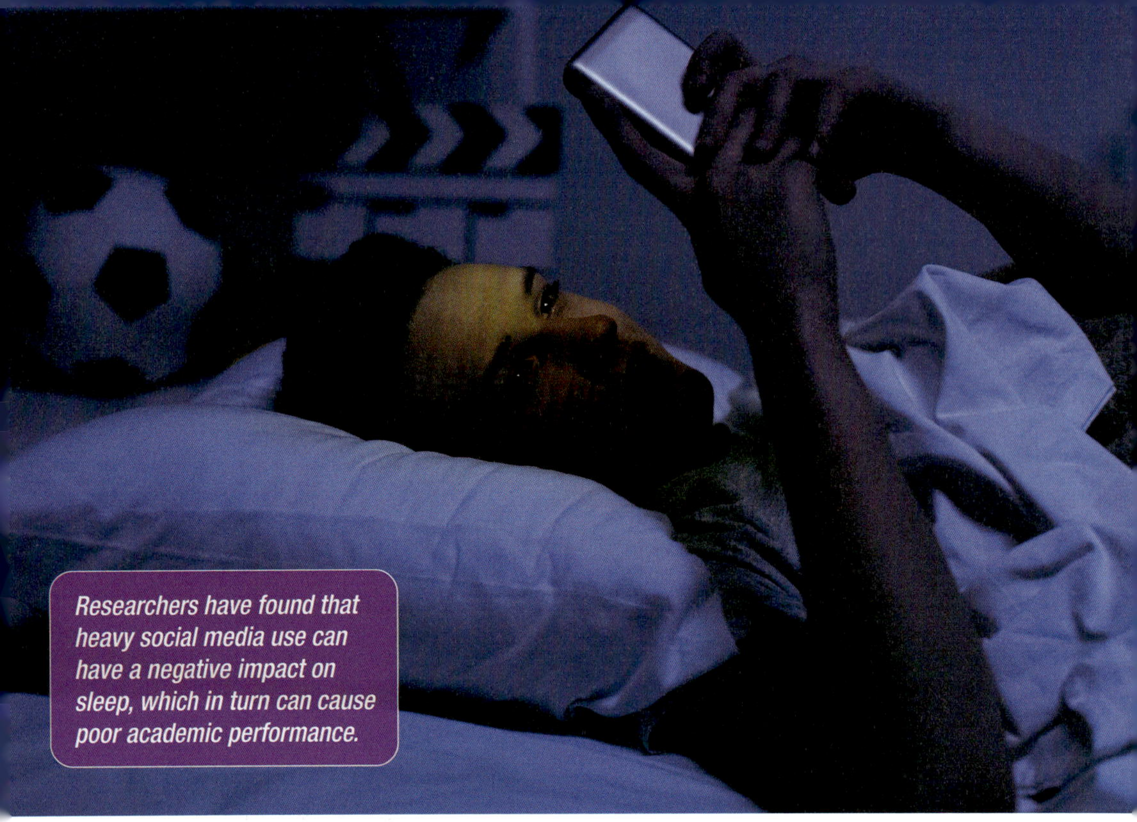

Researchers have found that heavy social media use can have a negative impact on sleep, which in turn can cause poor academic performance.

levels of anxiety and depression. Nighttime-specific social media use predicted poorer sleep quality even after taking into account other factors, including anxiety, depression, and self-esteem. The researchers wrote:

> These findings contribute to the growing body of evidence that social media use is related to various aspects of well-being in adolescents. In addition, our results indicate that nighttime-specific social media use and emotional investment in social media are two important factors that merit further investigation in relation to adolescent sleep and wellbeing.[35]

Depression

The University of Glasgow study is not the only one to find a link between problematic social media use and anxiety and depression. A 2018 study by researchers at the University of Pittsburgh

School of Medicine found a connection between the amount and intensity of social media use and elevated levels of anxiety and depression in adults. The researchers surveyed a nationally representative sample of 1,730 US adults aged nineteen to thirty-two, asking about their social media use and their mental health. The researchers divided the participants into five groups based on their social media use: "Wired," "Connected," "Diffuse Dabblers," "Concentrated Dabblers," and "Unplugged." The Wired and Connected groups spent the most time using social media and showed high emotional connection to the activity, including "a preoccupation with, and hyper-vigilant surveillance of, one's social media."[36] The members of these two groups who checked their social media most often showed elevated levels of depression compared to the general population. Members of the Unplugged, Concentrated Dabblers, and Diffuse Dabblers did not show increased levels of depression.

"I find myself, my mood and thoughts, influenced tremendously by scrolling mindlessly on social media platforms and by the content that I come across daily, even hourly."[37]

—A prelaw student who took part in a June 2018 Pew Research Center survey

A prelaw student who took part in a July 2018 Pew Research Center survey believes that social media is at the root of his depression. He says:

> I was recently diagnosed with mild depression. I believe that being hyperconnected within this digital life could be a root of the issue. I find myself, my mood and thoughts, influenced tremendously by scrolling mindlessly on social media platforms and by the content that I come across daily, even hourly. It has become increasingly hard to not constantly compare the reality of my life with those reflected through my iPhone screen and—even though I am aware of the false reality of the profiles I come across—it is hard not to have my own self-esteem and confidence plummet when I come across a perfectly tailored life.[37]

The Bergen Facebook Addiction Scale

Cecilie Schou Andreassen, professor at the Department of Clinical Psychology, University of Bergen, and her colleagues developed a six-question survey to distinguish between healthy and unhealthy Facebook use. Journalist Minu Budhia describes the survey:

- Those taking this test have to give one of the following five responses to each statement—Very rarely, Rarely, Sometimes, Often and Very often.
- You spend a lot of time thinking about Facebook or planning how to use it.
- You feel an urge to use Facebook more and more.
- You use Facebook in order to forget about personal problems.
- You have tried to cut down on the use of Facebook without success.
- You become restless or troubled if you are prohibited from using Facebook.
- You use Facebook so much that it has had a negative impact on your job/studies.
- Andreassen and her colleagues suggest that scoring 'Often' or 'Very often' on at least four of the six items may suggest the respondent is addicted to Facebook.

Minu Budhia, "How to Socialise Smartly," *Telegraph India*, July 6, 2019. www.telegraphindia.com.

The University of Pittsburgh study showed an association between social media use and depression, but it did not show that social media caused the depression. The researchers said that it was possible that the members of the Wired and Connected groups already had elevated levels of depression and their social media use only reflected those existing mental conditions. However, in December 2018, researchers at the University of Pennsylvania led by psychologist Melissa G. Hunt published a study that did show a causal link between social media use and depression.

In the University of Pennsylvania study, 143 students took a survey to measure their moods and mental well-being in several areas: social support, fear of missing out, loneliness, anxiety, depression, self-esteem, autonomy, and self-acceptance. The students were randomly divided into two groups. The students in one group maintained their typical social media behavior. This group was called the control group. The students in the other group were required to limit their time on Facebook, Snapchat, and Instagram to ten minutes per social media site per day for three weeks. This was called the experimental group. The researchers collected usage data from the participants' iPhones to verify that they followed the instructions. After three weeks, all of the participants took another survey. When the researchers compared the two surveys, they found that students who cut back their social media use reported decreases in loneliness and depression. The control group reported the same levels of depression and loneliness as before the experiment. "What we found overall is that if you use less social media, you are actually less depressed and less lonely, meaning that the decreased social media use is what causes that qualitative shift in your well-being," says Jordyn Young, a coauthor of the paper. "No matter where [the participants] started off, if they were told to limit their social media, they had less depression, no matter what their initial levels were."[38]

> "If you use less social media, you are actually less depressed and less lonely, meaning that the decreased social media use is what causes that qualitative shift in your well-being."[38]
>
> — Jordyn Young, researcher at the University of Pennsylvania

The University of Pennsylvania study did not attempt to explain why using social media causes depression, but Hunt believes that social media users feel bad about themselves because it appears that other people are leading better lives. "Some of the existing literature on social media suggests there's an enormous amount of social comparison that happens," says Hunt. "When you look at other people's lives, particularly on Instagram, it's easy to conclude that everyone else's life is cooler or better than yours."[39]

Brittany Smith, a digital marketing consultant based in North America, attests that she is affected by the comparisons she makes on social media.

> Overall, social media now takes away from my sense of well-being, and I try to limit my exposure to it. Initially, platforms such as Facebook helped me stay in touch with the people I care about. As more and more people joined Facebook and the algorithm changed I found that I was seeing less and less from them. Facebook was filled with updates from people who weren't close to me, and because of our tendency to share happy things that make us look good, I would come away feeling negative about my life.[40]

Another possible explanation for the improvement in well-being found in the University of Pennsylvania study is that cutting back on social media leaves more time for alternative, more positive activities and interactions. "When you're not busy getting sucked into clickbait social media, you're actually spending more time on things that are more likely to make you feel better about your life," says Hunt. "In general, I would say, put your phone down and be with the people in your life."[41]

Social Isolation

Most social media users visit social networking sites to connect with other people, but researchers at the University of Pittsburgh have found that young adults who use social media the most feel more socially isolated than those who use social media less. Heavy social media users reported a higher incidence of social isolation, a state in which an individual lacks a sense of social belonging, true engagement with others, and fulfilling relationships. Social isolation is a serious mental condition that has been associated with several negative health effects, including sleep disruption, impaired immune function, poor cognition, and an increased risk of mortality from all causes.

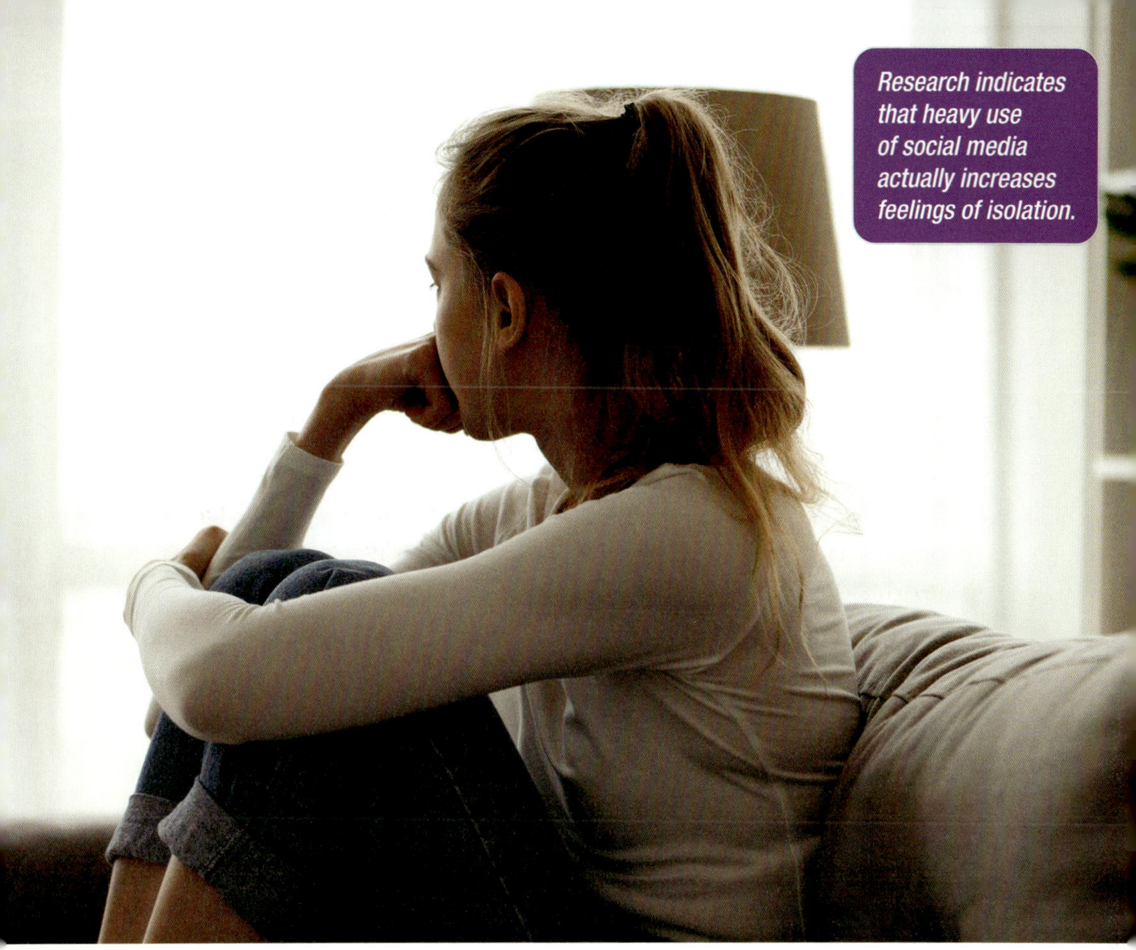

Research indicates that heavy use of social media actually increases feelings of isolation.

In a 2017 study, the University of Pittsburgh researchers surveyed 1,787 US adults aged nineteen to thirty-two years. They used standardized tests to measure the participants' social media use and their feelings of social isolation. For example, participants were asked how often in the past seven days they had feelings such as "I feel left out," "I feel that people barely know me," "I feel isolated from others," and "I feel that people are around me but not with me." The researchers found that the participants in the top 25 percent for time spent on social media were twice as likely to have greater perceived social isolation than those who ranked in the lowest 25 percent for time spent on social media. Similarly, those in the top 25 percent for the frequency of social media use were three times as likely to have greater perceived social isolation than those ranked in the lowest 25 percent for frequency of social media use.

The researchers saw two possible explanations for the increased feelings of social isolation. One possibility is that individuals who are already feeling socially isolated tend to use social media more. They may turn to social networks as a substitute for in-person social contact which they lack. The other possibility is that those who spend a lot of time on social media develop increased social isolation. This could be because the increased time spent on social media takes away from time spent in face-to-face communication. It is also possible that social media increases feelings of being excluded. "For example, an individual may discover pictures or other evidence of events to which they were not invited," write the researchers. This would increase feelings of being left out. Finally, heavy users of social media might be reacting to posts that are created to present the most positive events in peers' lives instead of representing reality. "Exposure to such highly idealized representations of peers' lives may elicit feelings of envy and the distorted belief that others lead happier and more successful lives, which may increase perceived social isolation,"[42] write the researchers. The researchers recommend further research to better understand reasons for the increased levels in social isolation.

Impaired Decision Making

Heavy use of social media also impairs decision-making, according to researchers at Michigan State University (MSU). The researchers administered a survey known as the Bergen Facebook Addiction Scale to seventy-one people to assess their involvement with Facebook. The survey included questions about how Facebook affected the participants' jobs or studies, how they felt when they were unable to use the site, and what happened when they tried to stop using the site. The researchers then had the participants perform one hundred trials of the Iowa Gambling Task (IGT), a psychological test designed to simulate real-life decision making. The MSU team found that the participants exhibiting the deepest emotional involvement with Facebook performed the worst on the decision-making test. "In particular, our results indicate that excessive users [of social networking sites] may make more risky decisions during the IGT task,"[43] write the researchers.

As revealed in other studies, the performance by excessive Facebook users was strikingly similar to that of people who are dependent on substances such as cocaine or heroin. "Decision making is oftentimes compromised in individuals with substance use disorders. They sometimes fail to learn from their mistakes and continue down a path of negative outcomes,"[44] explains Dar Meshi, an assistant professor in MSU's neuroscience program and leader of the MSU study. "Our research supports a parallel between individuals displaying problematic, excessive social media use and individuals with substance use disorders."[45]

"Our research supports a parallel between individuals displaying problematic, excessive social media use and individuals with substance use disorders."[45]

— Dar Meshi, assistant professor at Michigan State University

Physical Risks

Social media addiction not only affects the inner workings of the brain, but it also can affect the overall health of the body. Spending too much time looking at computers and cell phone screens has been shown to cause eye strain, neck pain, and lower back problems. A 2017 study by researchers at Queensland University in Australia found that people who use social media the most have "significantly greater sitting times while using a computer in leisure time and significantly greater total sitting time on non-workdays."[46] According to a 2017 study led by Keith Diaz, a researcher in the Columbia University Department of Medicine, sitting for long periods of time is linked to increased mortality. "Both the total volume of sedentary time and its accrual in prolonged, uninterrupted bouts are associated with all-cause mortality,"[47] wrote the researchers.

Excessive time spent on computers and other devices, for example, increases the risk of obesity. A 2017 study of high school students by researchers at the Harvard T.H. Chan School of Public Health in Boston found that using digital devices five hours a day or more was associated with increased consumption of sugary drinks, inadequate physical activity, and inadequate sleep. "Using smartphones, tablets, computers, and videogames is associated with several obesity risk factors,"[48] write the researchers.

A 2018 report from technology research firm GlobalWebIndex estimates that the global average for time spent on social media is two hours and twenty-two minutes per day. Those aged sixteen to twenty-four spend three hours a day on social media—that is just an average, however. A 2017 study by Eötvös Loránd University in Budapest, Hungary, found that problematic social media users spent 4.5 hours a day on social media, with some social media addicts spending even six hours daily. Those hours spent staring at screens, whether large or small, are producing eye strain, neck and shoulder pain, and disruptions in sleep patterns. The bombardment of social media notifications and the constant checking of social media websites are creating anxiety and even depression in users. "We have to start recognising the costs of time spent on social media," says Natasha Schüll, author of *Addiction by Design*. "It's not just a game—it affects us financially, physically and emotionally."[49]

Chapter Four

Treating Social Media Addiction

Addiction to substances like alcohol, cocaine, and heroin is usually treated by having the patient abstain from using any mood-altering chemical, because even a small dose can trigger a relapse into addiction. This approach is not practical for many behavioral addictions, including eating disorders, shopping addiction, and cell phone addiction, since activities associated with the addiction are necessary for life or nearly so. As a result, treatments for behavioral addiction often focus on modifying rather than eliminating the behavior.

While social media sites like Facebook and Twitter are not necessary for life, some online activities like emailing, texting, and video conferencing are required by many jobs and for modern life in general. As a result, social media addiction is often treated through behavior modification rather than by total abstinence. "The advantage of something like alcohol addiction is that you can stay away from bars; you can stay away from other drinkers; you can refrain from touching a drop of alcohol again," explains Hilarie Cash, the cofounder and chief clinical officer of technology addiction treatment center reSTART Life. "This is not that." Instead, social media addiction is similar to an eating disorder, because the patient will always be exposed to the source of their addiction. "Just as someone with an eating disorder has to learn how to avoid unhealthy foods that trigger their cycle, so, too, these clients have to learn to use the Internet in healthy ways and avoid things that will trigger their cycles,"[50] says Cash.

Technological Aids

At its most basic level, social media addiction is a dependence on technology: software applications, or apps, that enable social engagement online. As a result, technology is often enlisted to battle the addictions it has spawned. Many software developers have created apps that help users to modify online behavior. Some apps allow the user to block access to specific websites, including social media websites. For some social media addicts, website blocking and their own determination to quit is enough to end their excessive social networking activity.

> **"Just as someone with an eating disorder has to learn how to avoid unhealthy foods that trigger their cycle, so, too, these clients have to learn to use the Internet in healthy ways and avoid things that will trigger their cycles."[50]**
>
> —Hilarie Cash, cofounder and chief clinical officer of technology addiction treatment center reSTART Life

Other software programs allow users to limit the amount of time they can spend each day on a social media website. For example, the user might set a limit of ten minutes on a social media site—just enough time to check messages and respond to the most urgent ones, or even to post an important announcement. These apps often maintain a record of online activity. Social media users can use these logs as a tool to keep themselves accountable for their behavior. They can also share the information with a relative, friend, or therapist who is helping the user overcome the addiction.

Professional Treatment

Dependence on social media is sometimes so intense that do-it-yourself methods do not work. Some social media addicts need face-to-face counseling with an addiction counselor, a psychotherapist, or a psychiatrist. Some can be helped with group therapy, meeting with their peers to learn coping techniques and to gain emotional support for their recovery. Others may need medical intervention, including treatment with medication.

One of the most common treatments for social media addiction is cognitive behavioral therapy (CBT). This therapy addresses the process of thinking, known as cognition. The CBT counselor, usually a psychologist or a mental health therapist, meets one-on-one with the patient. Usually these meetings are in-person, but some counselors now provide treatment online. During these sessions, the counselor works with the patient to identify the thought processes that lead to the harmful behavior, in this case going online and engaging with social media. The patient learns to notice these thoughts as they occur and then pause before acting on them. The counselor also gives the patient strategies

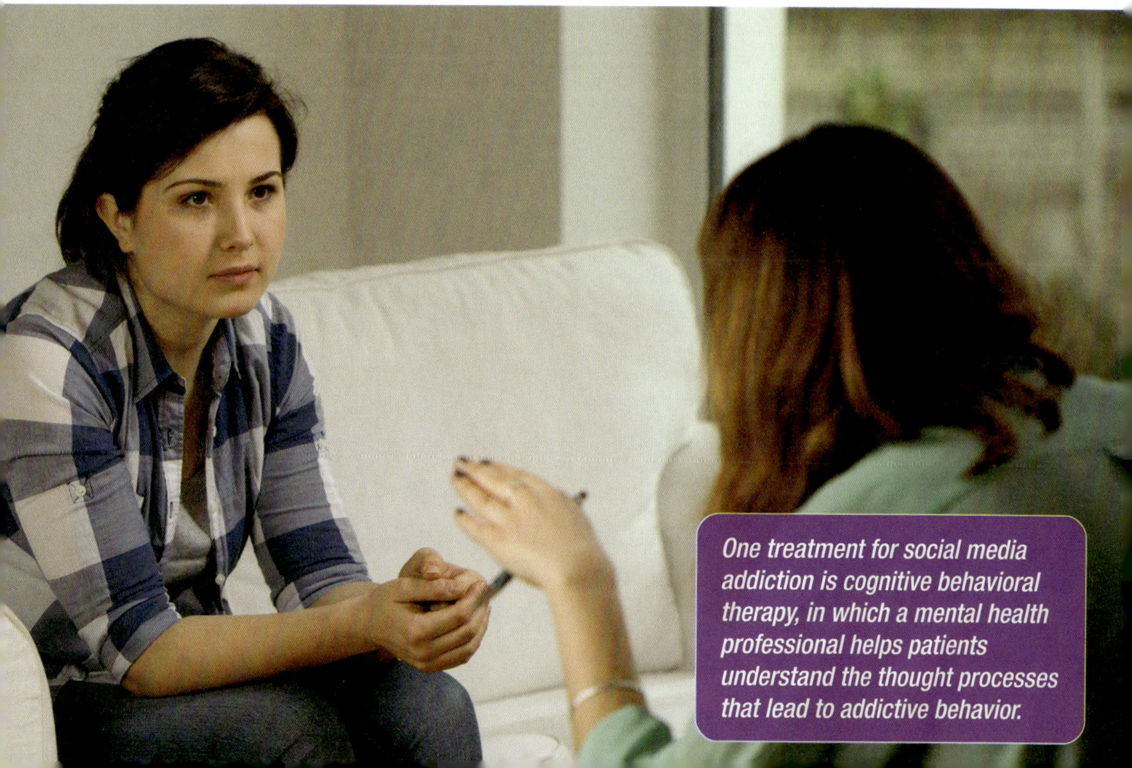

One treatment for social media addiction is cognitive behavioral therapy, in which a mental health professional helps patients understand the thought processes that lead to addictive behavior.

to challenge and overcome their addiction-related thoughts, thus preventing the addictive behavior.

CBT is often successful because it focuses directly on the addictive behavior. However, the impulse to engage in social media may spring from deeper psychological issues. Unless these issues are addressed, the patient will continue to exhibit addictive behavior. He or she might stop using social media but then switch to another destructive behavior—gaming addiction, gambling addiction, or even substance addiction. For example, the patient may be suffering from anxiety or depression related to physical abuse, sexual abuse, or another trauma. In such cases, the patient needs to address the underlying issues with a psychotherapist, psychiatrist, or other mental health professional. Says therapist Nicole Amesbury:

> As therapists we see problems, all the time, every day, with someone coming in, and as they're telling us about what they're struggling with, they'll bring up a social media piece. But some people don't think of that being a part of their overall mental health. When people come to therapy, they usually come with a thing that they need to work on—a relationship, a habit, a fear—and they pop it in there and say, this is my problem, and it seems very well defined. But of course, you're a whole person.[51]

In some cases, the underlying psychological issues may involve other family members. There may be tensions within the home that are affecting everyone's behavior and contributing to the social media addiction. Unless the family dynamics are addressed, the addiction treatment might not be effective. In these situations, the whole family may undergo treatment as a group, a process known as family therapy. "Family therapy views a person's symptoms as taking place in the larger context of the family," writes psychologist Michael Herkov. "Without understanding that larger group and the complex, dynamic interactions that take

A Seventeen-Year-Old Social Media Addict Quits

Corey Simon, a self-described social media addict, closed all of his social media accounts at once.

> Social media. The time wasting, addictive drugs that let us subliminally express our deepest narcissistic thoughts. At least, that's how I saw them. Maybe your situation is different. Like any powerful tool, social media can be used for good, as well as bad—and in my particular case, it was bad.
>
> It's safe to say while I was addicted to social media, I was disconnected from the real world. Not only was I spending most of my spare time on it, but when I was engaging in real life social interactions I wasn't really "present." I was more focused on scrolling through my Facebook newsfeed. Ironically, I remember thinking, "If I delete all my social media, won't I turn into one of those disconnected, weird people who never leave their room?"—which is essentially what I was, while thinking that. Funny.
>
> Deleting social media has been the best decision I have ever made. It's made me closer to my family, more disciplined towards my studies, eat healthier, work out more and has given me plenty of free time to read as many books as I'd like. Life is great.

Corey Simon, "I'm 17 and I Deleted All My Social Media. Here's What Happened," *Medium*, April 30, 2017. https://medium.com.

place and how those interactions were formed, it may not be as easy to help the identified patient (the person with the 'problem' that everyone else in the family is concerned about)."[52]

In family therapy, the therapist identifies patterns of behavior within the family and how these patterns contribute to the behavioral addiction. For example, a family member might be using social media as an escape from other problems in the household, such as arguing or emotional abuse, or as a response to a medical crisis or death in the family. After identifying negative patterns in the family, the therapist creates a plan to change them. The therapist works with family members to improve communication and identify and solve problems, creating a healthier home environment. Addressing these underlying issues improves the chances that the addiction treatment will be successful.

Accompanying Disorders

Sometimes the underlying problem contributing to social media addiction is one of mental health. Since social media addiction and the underlying disorder are often linked, a social media addict may need dual diagnosis treatment—treatment that addresses both the addiction and some degree of mental illness. Dual diagnosis treatment allows the medical professional to find the root cause of the behavior and determine the best treatment.

Substance addiction is another disorder that can accompany social media addiction. Like an underlying mental disorder, substance abuse can affect impulse control and lead to excessive use of social media. Sometimes alcohol or drug abuse is secret, and excessive social media use is the visible symptom of the accompanying addiction. If a person has both a substance addiction and a behavioral addiction, both must be treated at the same time.

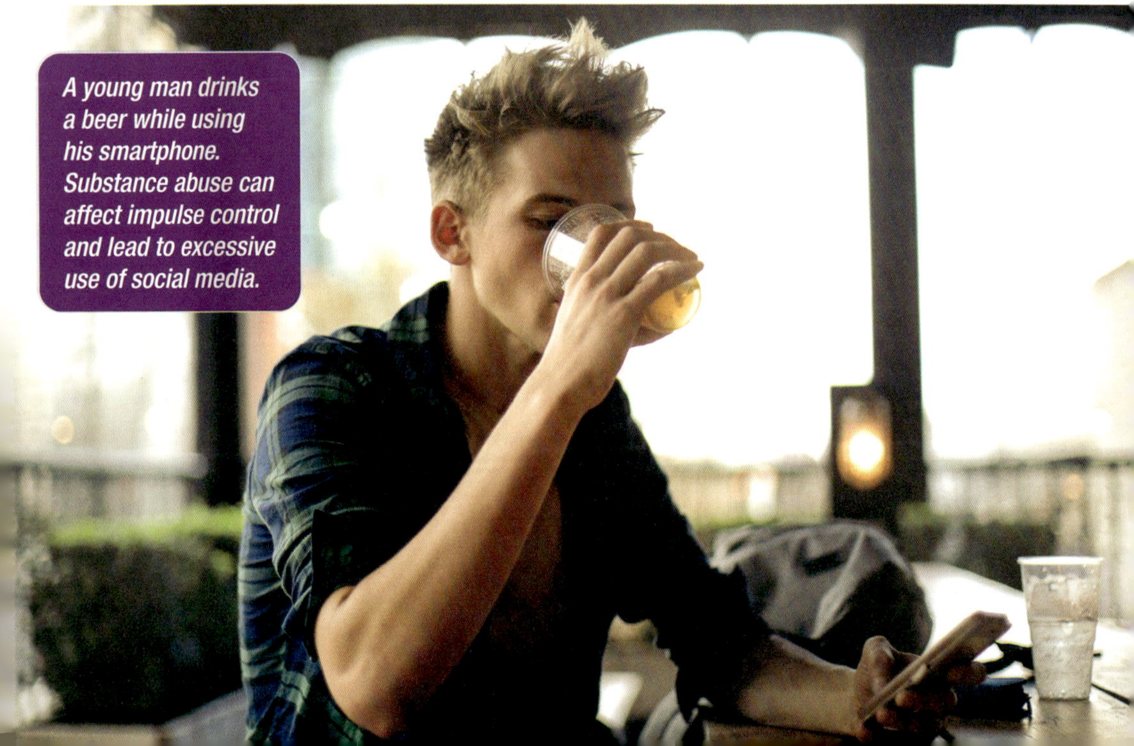

A young man drinks a beer while using his smartphone. Substance abuse can affect impulse control and lead to excessive use of social media.

Twelve-Step Programs

Some organizations treat gaming addiction using a twelve-step program similar to the one pioneered by the alcoholism treatment organization Alcoholics Anonymous. The success of the twelve-step approach in treating alcoholism has led others to adopt the program for different addictions. Among the organizations treating addiction with this method are Narcotics Anonymous, Nicotine Anonymous, Overeaters Anonymous, and Gamblers Anonymous. Social media addiction is also being treated in twelve-step programs, sometimes by itself and sometimes along with other technological addictions, such as internet addiction and gaming addiction.

In twelve-step programs, the person with the addiction meets with a group of people who are also addicted. This arrangement is known as a peer-to-peer model of treatment. Outsiders are not allowed into the meetings. This is an important aspect of the treatment. All of the people in the room share the same struggle. They know what the addiction is like, how it forms, and all of the excuses that people make to continue their addiction.

The members use only their first names, so they can remain anonymous. In addition, all members promise to keep what is said in the meetings private. Because of these safeguards, the people in the group can be completely honest about their addiction without fear of damaging their reputation. They are encouraged to tell their addiction story. In return, other members share their stories, both to show support and to provide encouragement and guidance for the person seeking help. "As opposed to giving advice, the recovery community shares with one another what worked for them [in] similar situations," states the blog of the PACE Recovery Center, a twelve-step treatment center in Orange County, California. "It is a method that does not make one feel admonished or patronized. On the other hand, you feel as though you are a part of something greater than yourself. A part of a fellowship that has a vested interest in your success."[53]

> **"As opposed to giving advice, the recovery community shares with one another what worked for them [in] similar situations."[53]**
>
> — PACE Recovery Center blog

Twelve-step programs also pair each recovering addict with a more experienced person who is also in recovery, known as a sponsor. The sponsor helps the recovering addict work their way through the twelve steps of the recovery program. The sponsor is available around the clock to speak with the recovering addict any time that person is considering going back to the addictive behavior.

A young tech worker in Seattle credits his sponsor with helping him battle his technology addiction. "He's a role model," the young man says of his sponsor, Charlie. "He has a place of his own. He has a dog. He has friends." The young man tried to quit on his own, even convincing his mother to get rid of the home Wi-Fi system to reduce the temptation of going online. Despite these precautions, he would still relapse. "Then, I discover very quickly that I am actually an addict," he says. With Charlie's guidance, he realizes he needs to continue to work the twelve-step program. "I do need to do this,"[54] he says. Now, he has put apps on his phone that send reports about his online activity to Charlie.

Treatment Centers

Sometimes a behavioral addiction is so severe that meeting with counselors or twelve-step groups is not enough to break the pattern of destructive behavior. In such cases, addicts can benefit from leaving their home environment and entering a residential treatment program. This is a facility where an addict can live with others struggling with addiction, isolated from the substance or, in the case of a social media addiction, the technology behind the addiction. This disruption of the addict's everyday life helps to break the pattern of the addiction. It also brings the addict in contact with other addicts who are facing the same struggle, as in a twelve-step program. The presence of these peers helps the patient feel understood and supported. Such centers also offer addiction counseling, both for individuals and in groups.

Because social media addiction is relatively new, there are few residential treatment centers dedicated solely to treating social

Leaving Social Media for Audiobooks

Michael Cappetta, a television producer for NBC News, tells how audiobooks helped him kick his social media habit.

> When Apple released the "Time Spent" feature in a recent iOS update, I was absolutely disgusted by the wasted hours I had logged endlessly scrolling through Instagram, Facebook, LinkedIn, Twitter and Snap. . . .
>
> Earlier this year, a friend suggested I start listening to audiobooks. I initially disregarded the idea, thinking it may be tough to start/stop books on the go. . . . Despite my objections, my friend convinced me to give it a try.
>
> The next morning on my commute to work, I listened to the audiobook for about 30 minutes. At first, it was a tough adjustment. My natural reflex whenever my subway stopped was to pull up Twitter and start scrolling for updates. This time, I was pulled into the narrative and kept my phone in my pocket. The audiobooks had become a welcome distraction from the constant buzz of social media. . . .
>
> Since adopting these new strategies, and by moving social media apps off of my home screen, I have reduced my time spent on social media by 85 percent.

Michael Cappetta, "The App That Helped Me Quit My Social Media Addiction," NBC News, April 24, 2019. www.nbcnews.com.

media addiction. As a result, social media addicts often receive treatment at centers for other behavioral addictions, including technology addiction and gambling addiction. One of these is reSTART Life, a residential treatment center outside Seattle, Washington. Founded by Hilarie Cash and Cosette Rae, a former software developer, reSTART Life provides a way for social media and technology addicts to remove themselves from all of the internet temptations of work and home for a period from eight weeks to twelve months. The residents are allowed to have cell phones, but they can only use them to communicate with friends and family, not to browse the web. The residents not only work on their mental state but also on their bodies. Junk food is banned. Residents are served healthy food and are required to take part in an exercise program. To overcome sleep deprivation, residents must adhere to a strict sleep schedule. The residents receive individual and group counseling and must make a "bottom line" promise to give up their problem behavior. "I came into this program because I figured that I would either have to change, or I would just end up killing myself," says Jason Klinkman, twenty-three. "It's like any other addiction where you shut out the feelings and then the feelings get worse and worse. It can lead you down to very dark places."[55] At the end of their treatment, residents are encouraged to look for employment or return to school. "This is a much-needed resource for families," says Rae, who is also the CEO of reSTART Life. "The need is great and availability is scarce, but hope and understanding are in no short supply. Our office has received thousands of calls from parents over the years and the ages of children who need help are continually getting younger. These children are choosing to step out of life and into their device."[56]

> **"[Residential treatment centers are] a much-needed resource for families. The need is great and availability is scarce, but hope and understanding are in no short supply."[56]**
>
> — Cosette Rae, cofounder and CEO of reSTART Life

Governmental Intervention

Some political leaders believe government has a role in reducing social media addiction. Senator Joshua "Josh" Hawley, a Republican from Missouri, believes Congress should ban certain practices that feed social media addiction. "Big Tech has embraced addiction as a business model," Hawley tweeted in July 2019. "Their 'innovation' isn't designed to create better products, but to capture attention by using psychological tricks that make it impossible to look away. Time to expect more & better from Silicon Valley."[57]

Hawley introduced a bill in the Senate that addresses social media practices head-on. The bill states that its purpose is to "prohibit social media companies from using practices that exploit human psychology or brain physiology to substantially impede freedom of choice, to require social media companies to take measures to mitigate the risks of internet addiction and psychological exploitation, and for other purposes."[58]

The bill targets several industry practices. One is infinite scroll or auto refill, a software feature that automatically loads new content into the Facebook newsfeed or a Twitter timeline without requiring any specific request from the user. These features make it possible for users to scroll through their social media feeds for hours on end. The bill requires social media platforms to include natural stopping points to prevent endless scrolling. Another banned feature is autoplay, a function that plays videos or music automatically. In particular, the bill forbids advertisements from playing automatically as people scroll through their feeds. There are exceptions to the autoplay ban that would allow users to stream music or play the user's music or video

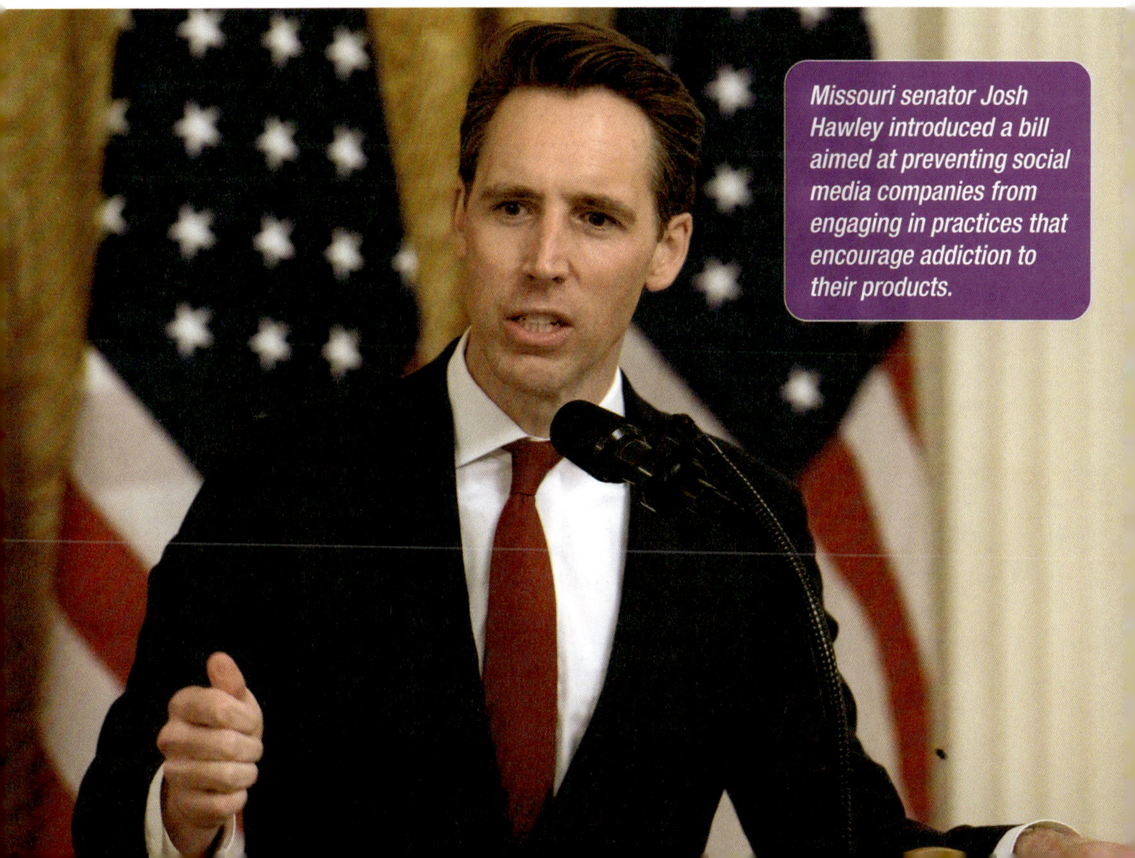

Missouri senator Josh Hawley introduced a bill aimed at preventing social media companies from engaging in practices that encourage addiction to their products.

playlist. The bill forbids sites and apps from providing users with badges and other awards for engaging with the social media. For example, the photo-sharing social media platform Snapchat awards "Snapstreak" badges in recognition of how long two friends have exchanged daily messages. Critics believe that Snapstreak badges exert undue pressure on young people to keep such streaks alive by using the app every day. It also requires social media companies to provide a tool within the app that enables users to track the amount of time they spend on social media across all devices and to impose caps on the time they spend using the social media platform. The bill was referred to committee for further study.

Finding Alternatives to Social Networking

For social media addicts, social networking replaces other leisure activities that they might have enjoyed before becoming preoccupied with social media. As a result, when an addict gives up social media, he or she will have a lot of free time. To avoid relapse, the recovering social media addict is encouraged to fill the free time with other activities, either returning to hobbies or finding new ones. "I needed to replace my social media habit with something else," says Anthony Pacheco, a digital marketing specialist. "So I started reading on my phone, as opposed to checking my Snapchat, scrolling through Facebook to see what my 'friends' were up to, browsing through Instagram, or [scrolling] through Twitter and [retweeting] today's nonsense."[59]

Social media affects everyone differently, and treatment for social media addiction can take many forms. Some people have found it a habit that can simply be changed by replacing it with another activity that produces less anxiety. Others need the guidance of a counselor or therapist to redirect their thoughts using cognitive behavior therapy. Those with underlying mental conditions may need intense individual therapy. In the most severe cases, the social media addict might need to disconnect from technology completely by enrolling in a residential treatment center.

Introduction: A Crisis in the Making

1. Chrissa Hardy, "I'm Addicted to Social Media & It's Ruining My Life," *Bolde*, February 24, 2017. www.bolde.com.
2. Hardy, "I'm Addicted to Social Media & It's Ruining My Life."

Chapter One: The Scope of Social Media Addiction

3. Carrie Battan, "How to Escape the Seduction of Your Smartphone," *Harper's Bazaar*, July 27, 2018. www.harpersbazaar.com.
4. Quoted in Chuck Hadad, "Why Some 13-Year-Olds Check Social Media 100 Times a Day," CNN, October 13, 2015. https://edition.cnn.com.
5. Cecilie Schou Andreassen, Ståle Pallesen, and Mark D. Griffiths, "The Relationship Between Addictive Use of Social Media, Narcissism, and Self-Esteem: Findings from a Large National Survey," *Addictive Behaviors*, March 19, 2016. http://iranarze.ir.
6. Quoted in Hadad, "Why Some 13-Year-Olds Check Social Media 100 Times a Day."
7. Marcello Russo, Massimo Bergami, and Gabriele Morandin, "Surviving a Day Without Smartphones," *MIT Sloan Management Review*, Winter 2018, pp. 8–9. www.mitsmr-ezine.com.
8. Quoted in Sabrina Tavernise, "Young Adolescents as Likely to Die from Suicide as from Traffic Accidents," *New York Times*, November 3, 2016. www.nytimes.com.
9. Quoted in Hadad, "Why Some 13-Year-Olds Check Social Media 100 Times a Day."
10. Quoted in Jean M. Twenge, "Have Smartphones Destroyed a Generation?," *The Atlantic*, September 2017. www.theatlantic.com.
11. Andreassen, Pallesen, and Griffiths, "The Relationship Between Addictive Use of Social Media, Narcissism, and Self-Esteem."

12. Cecilie Schou Andreassen, "Online Social Network Site Addiction: A Comprehensive Review," *Current Addiction Reports*, June 2015. https://link.springer.com.
13. Lancaster University, "Social Media Stress Can Lead to Social Media Addiction," *Science Daily*, August 27, 2019. www.sciencedaily.com.
14. Lancaster University, "Social Media Stress Can Lead to Social Media Addiction."
15. Quoted in Eduardo Guedes et al., "Internet Addiction and Excessive Social Networks Use: What About Facebook?," *Clinical Practices in Epidemiological Mental Health*, June 28, 2016. www.ncbi.nlm.nih.gov.
16. Quoted in Kelly Wallace, "Half of Teens Think They're Addicted to Their Smartphones," CNN, July 29, 2016. http://edition.cnn.com.

Chapter Two: Why People Become Addicted to Social Media

17. "Reality Behind the Claims of Social Media Addiction," *Digital Information World*, July 11, 2018. www.digitalinformationworld.com.
18. Quoted in Chloe Metzger, "I'm in Love with Myself: The Age of Digital Narcissism," *Marie Claire*, February 12, 2018. www.marieclaire.com.
19. Quoted in Paul Lewis, "'Our Minds Can Be Hijacked': The Tech Insiders Who Fear a Smartphone Dystopia," *The Guardian*, December 12, 2017. www.theguardian.com.
20. Quoted in Mattha Busby, "Social Media Copies Gambling Methods 'to Create Psychological Cravings,'" *The Guardian*, May 8, 2018. www.theguardian.com.
21. Quoted in Busby, "Social Media Copies Gambling Methods 'to Create Psychological Cravings.'"
22. Shaun Smith, "My Social Media Addiction," *Daddy's Digest*, February 18, 2019. https://daddysdigest.com.
23. Smith, "My Social Media Addiction."
24. Smith, "My Social Media Addiction."
25. Smith, "My Social Media Addiction."
26. Quoted in Lewis, "'Our Minds Can Be Hijacked.'"
27. "Reality Behind the Claims of Social Media Addiction."
28. Quoted in Janna Anderson and Lee Rainie, "Stories from Experts About the Impact of Digital Life," *Pew Research*, July 3, 2018. www.pewinternet.org.
29. Jane E. Brody, "Hooked on Our Smartphones," *New York Times*, January 9, 2017. www.nytimes.com.

30. Quoted in Busby, "Social Media Copies Gambling Methods 'to Create Psychological Cravings.'"
31. Quoted in Gigen Mammoser, "The FOMO Is Real: How Social Media Increases Depression and Loneliness," Healthline. www.healthline.com.
32. Quoted in Megan Teske, "Iowa State Research Shows That Some May Be at More Risk for Video Game Addiction," *Iowa State Daily*, November 6, 2018. www.iowastatedaily.com.

Chapter Three: The Effects of Social Media Addiction

33. Quoted in "Problematic Social Media Use Linked to Brain Imbalance," *Science Direct*, March 15, 2017. www.sciencedaily.com.
34. Holly Scott and Heather Cleland Woods, "Fear of Missing Out and Sleep: Cognitive Behavioural Factors in Adolescents' Nighttime Social Media Use," *Journal of Adolescence*, October 2018. www.ncbi.nlm.nih.gov.
35. Holly Scott and Heather Cleland Woods, "#Sleepyteens: Social Media Use in Adolescence Is Associated with Poor Sleep Quality, Anxiety, Depression and Low Self-Esteem," *Journal of Adolescence*, August 2016.
36. Ariel Shensa et al., "Social Media Use and Depression and Anxiety Symptoms: A Cluster Analysis," *American Journal of Health Behavior*, March 1, 2018. www.ncbi.nlm.nih.gov.
37. Quoted in Janna Anderson and Lee Rainie, "Stories from Experts About the Impact of Digital Life," *Pew Research*, July 3, 2018. www.pewinternet.org.
38. Quoted in Gigen Mammoser, "The FOMO Is Real: How Social Media Increases Depression and Loneliness," *Healthline*, December 9, 2018. www.healthline.com.
39. Quoted in University of Pennsylvania, "Social Media Use Increases Depression and Loneliness, Study Finds," *Science News*, November 8, 2018. www.sciencedaily.com.
40. Quoted in Anderson and Rainie, "Stories from Experts About the Impact of Digital Life."
41. Quoted in University of Pennsylvania, "Social Media Use Increases Depression and Loneliness."
42. Brian A. Primack et al., "Social Media Use and Perceived Social Isolation Among Young Adults in the U.S.," *American Journal of Preventative Medicine*, July 2017. www.ncbi.nlm.nih.gov.
43. Dar Meshi et al., "Excessive Social Media Users Demonstrate Impaired Decision Making in the Iowa Gambling Task," *Journal of Behavioral Addictions*, March 1, 2019. www.ncbi.nlm.nih.gov.

44. Quoted in Caroline Brooks, "Excessive Social Media Use Is Comparable to Drug Addiction," *MSU Today*, January 10, 2019. https://msutoday.msu.edu.
45. Dar Meshi, interview with the author, September 9, 2019.
46. Stephanie Jade Alley et al., "Impact of Increasing Social Media Use on Sitting Time and Body Mass Index," *Health Promotion Journal of Australia*, August 28, 2017. www.ncbi.nlm.nih.gov.
47. Keith Diaz et al., "Patterns of Sedentary Behavior and Mortality in U.S. Middle-Aged and Older Adults: A National Cohort Study," *Annals of Internal Medicine*, October 3, 2017. www.ncbi.nlm.nih.gov.
48. Erica Kenney and Steven Gortmaker, "United States Adolescents' Television, Computer, Videogame, Smartphone, and Tablet Use: Associations with Sugary Drinks, Sleep, Physical Activity, and Obesity," *Journal of Pediatrics*, March 2017. www.ncbi.nlm.nih.gov.
49. Quoted in Busby, "Social Media Copies Gambling Methods 'to Create Psychological Cravings.'"

Chapter Four: Treating Social Media Addiction

50. Quoted in Molly Young, "What an Internet Rehabilitation Program Is Really Like," *Allure*, January 21, 2018. www.allure.com.
51. Quoted in Sarah Kessler, "What I Learned in 12 Weeks of Therapy for Social Media Addiction," *Fast Company*, January 8, 2016. www.fastcompany.com.
52. Michael Herkov, "About Family Therapy," *Psych Central*, October 8, 2018. https://psychcentral.com.
53. "Addiction Recovery: Peer-to-Peer Model," PACE Recovery Center blog, August 23, 2017. www.pacerecoverycenter.com.
54. Quoted in Associated Press, "'Tech Addicts' Seek Solace in 12 Steps and Rehab," *Tampa Bay Times* (St. Petersburg, FL), December 26, 2018. www.tampabay.com.
55. Quoted in Stephen Cohen, "Rehab Center Treats Internet Addicts in Microsoft's Backyard," *SeattlePI*, February 20, 2018. www.seattlepi.com.
56. "reSTART Opens First Internet Videogame Addiction Center for Youth in US," *Cision*, November 17, 2016. www.prweb.com.
57. Josh Hawley (@HawleyMO), "Big Tech has embraced addiction as a business model," Twitter, July 30, 2019. https://twitter.com/HawleyMO/status/1156203526688841728.
58. Joshua Hawley, "The Social Media Addiction Reduction Technology (SMART) Act," *Josh Hawley*, July 30, 2019. www.hawley.senate.gov.
59. Anthony Pacheco, "How Social Media Is Important to My Job, but Shouldn't Be Important to My Life," *Medium*, September 6, 2019. https://medium.com.

Center for Safe and Responsible Internet Use—www.cyberbully.org

The Center for Safe and Responsible Internet Use helps young people keep themselves safe and respect others on the internet. Its website contains information designed to help people learn about responsible internet behavior.

Childnet International—www.childnet.com

Childnet International's mission is to work in partnership with others around the world to help make the internet a safe place for children. Its website features news; projects; general safety advice for parents, young people, and teachers; links; and other information.

Common Sense Media—www.commonsensemedia.org

Common Sense Media is an independent nonprofit organization that provides education, ratings, and tools to families to promote safe technology and media for children and teens. Its goal is to help kids thrive in a world of media and technology.

Get Net Wise—www.getnetwise.org

Get Net Wise is a website provided by internet industry corporations and public interest organizations. Its goal is to ensure that internet users have safe and constructive online experiences. The website contains information about youth safety, security, and privacy.

Pew Research Center—http://pewinternet.org

Through its Pew Internet & American Life Project, the center studies how Americans use the internet and how digital technologies are shaping the world today. Its website has the results of numerous studies about privacy and the internet.

Stay Safe Online—www.staysafeonline.org

Part of the National Cyber Security Alliance, this website offers educational materials, information for home users on protecting their computers and their children, cybersecurity practices, videos, a self-assessment quiz, and additional information.

Books

Adam Alter, *Irresistible: The Rise of Addictive Technology and the Business of Keeping Us Hooked*. New York: Penguin Press, 2018.

Mark Carrier, *From Smartphones to Social Media: How Technology Affects Our Brains and Behavior.* Santa Barbara, CA: Greenwood, 2018.

Nicholas Kardaras, *Glow Kids: How Screen Addiction Is Hijacking Our Kids—and How to Break the Trance*. New York: St. Martin's Griffin, 2017.

Jaron Lanier, *Ten Arguments For Deleting Your Social Media Accounts Right Now*. New York: Henry Holt, 2018.

Peggy J. Parks, *Social Media*. San Diego: ReferencePoint Press, 2017.

Bradley Steffens, *Cell Phone Addiction*. San Diego: ReferencePoint Press, 2020.

Jean M. Twenge, *iGen: Why Today's Super-Connected Kids Are Growing Up Less Rebellious, More Tolerant, Less Happy—and Completely Unprepared for Adulthood*. New York: Atria, 2017.

Internet Sources

Janna Anderson and Lee Rainie, "Stories from Experts About the Impact of Digital Life," *Pew Research*, July 3, 2018. www.pewinternet.org.

Daniel Kruger, "Social Media Copies Gambling Methods 'to Create Psychological Cravings,'" *Institute for Healthcare Policy & Innovation*, May 8, 2018. https://ihpi.umich.edu.

Chloe Metzger, "I'm in Love with Myself: The Age of Digital Narcissism," *Marie Claire*, February 12, 2018. www.marieclaire.com.

Gigen Mammoser, "The FOMO Is Real: How Social Media Increases Depression and Loneliness," *Healthline*, December 9, 2018. www.healthline.com.

Simon Parkin, "Has Dopamine Got Us Hooked on Tech?," *The Guardian* (US edition), March 4, 2018. www.theguardian.com.

Molly Young, "What an Internet Rehabilitation Program Is Really Like," *Allure*, January 21, 2018. www.allure.com.